Melanoma

Editors

KEITH A. DELMAN
MICHAEL C. LOWE

SURGICAL ONCOLOGY CLINICS OF NORTH AMERICA

www.surgonc.theclinics.com

Consulting Editor
TIMOTHY M. PAWLIK

July 2020 • Volume 29 • Number 3

ELSEVIER

1600 John F. Kennedy Boulevard • Suite 1800 • Philadelphia, Pennsylvania, 19103-2899

http://www.theclinics.com

SURGICAL ONCOLOGY CLINICS OF NORTH AMERICA Volume 29, Number 3
July 2020 ISSN 1055-3207, ISBN-13: 978-0-323-72082-3

Editor: John Vassallo (j.vassallo@elsevier.com)
Developmental Editor: Julia Mckenzie

Surgical Oncology Clinics of North America (ISSN 1055-3207) is published quarterly by Elsevier Inc., 360 Park Avenue South, New York, NY 10010-1710. Months of publication are January, April, July, and October. Business and Editorial Offices: 1600 John F. Kennedy Blvd., Ste. 1800, Philadelphia, PA 19103-2899. Customer Service Office: 3251 Riverport Lane, Maryland Heights, MO 63043. Periodicals postage paid at New York, NY and additional mailing offices. Subscription prices are $309.00 per year (US individuals), $562.00 (US institutions) $100.00 (US student/resident), $352.00 (Canadian individuals), $711.00 (Canadian institutions), $100.00 (Canadian student/resident), $422.00 (foreign individuals), $711.00 (foreign institutions), and $205.00 (foreign student/resident). Foreign air speed delivery is included in all *Clinics* subscription prices. All prices are subject to change without notice. **POSTMASTER**: Send address changes to *Surgical Oncology Clinics of North America*, Elsevier Health Science Division, Subscription Customer Service, 3251 Riverport Lane, Maryland Heights, MO 63043. **Customer Service: 1-800-654-2452 (US and Canada). 314-447-8871 (outside US and Canada). Fax: 314-447-8029. E-mail: journalscustomerservice-usa@elsevier.com (for print support); journalsonline support-usa@elsevier.com (for online support).**

Reprints. For copies of 100 or more, of articles in this publication, please contact the Commercial Reprints Department, Elsevier Inc., 360 Park Avenue South, New York, New York 10010-1710. Tel. 212-633-3874; Fax: 212-633-3820; E-mail: reprints@elsevier.com.

Surgical Oncology Clinics of North America is covered in *MEDLINE/PubMed (Index Medicus)* and *EMBASE/ Excerpta Medica, Current Contents/Clinical Medicine,* and *ISI/BIOMED.*

Contributors

CONSULTING EDITOR

TIMOTHY M. PAWLIK, MD, MPH, PhD, FACS, FRACS (Hon.)
Professor and Chair, Department of Surgery, The Urban Meyer III and Shelley Meyer Chair for Cancer Research, Professor of Surgery, Oncology, Health Services Management and Policy, The Ohio State University, Wexner Medical Center, Columbus, Ohio

EDITORS

KEITH A. DELMAN, MD, FACS
Carlos Professor of Surgery, Division of Surgical Oncology, Department of Surgery, Winship Cancer Institute of Emory University School of Medicine, Atlanta, Georgia

MICHAEL C. LOWE, MD, MA, FACS
Assistant Professor of Surgery, Division of Surgical Oncology, Department of Surgery, Winship Cancer Institute of Emory University School of Medicine, Atlanta, Georgia

AUTHORS

CHRISTINA V. ANGELES, MD
Department of Surgery, University of Michigan, Ann Arbor, Michigan

EDMUND K. BARTLETT, MD
Assistant Attending Surgeon, Department of Surgery, Memorial Sloan Kettering Cancer Center, New York, New York

GEORGIA M. BEASLEY, MD, MHS
Department of Surgery, Duke University, Durham, North Carolina

ADAM C. BERGER, MD
Chief of Melanoma and Soft Tissue Oncology, Cancer Institute of New Jersey, New Brunswick, New Jersey

RUSSELL S. BERMAN, MD, FACS
Associate Professor, Department of Surgery, NYU Langone Health, New York, New York

EMMA BRADLEY, BS
Department of Surgery, Sidney Kimmel Medical College, Thomas Jefferson University, Philadelphia, Pennsylvania

KLAUS J. BUSAM, MD
Attending Pathologist, Department of Pathology, Memorial Sloan Kettering Cancer Center, New York, New York

CARRIE K. CHU, MD, MS, FACS
Department of Plastic Surgery, The University of Texas M.D. Anderson Cancer Center, Houston, Texas

JOSEPH G. CROMPTON, MD, PhD
Fellow Surgeon, Department of Surgery, Memorial Sloan Kettering Cancer Center, New York, New York

JESSICA CRYSTAL, MD
Complex General Surgical Oncology Fellow, Cedars-Sinai Medical Center, Los Angeles, California

MICHAEL E. EGGER, MD, MPH
Assistant Professor, The Hiram C. Polk Jr., MD, Department of Surgery, University of Louisville, Louisville, Kentucky

MARK B. FARIES, MD, FACS
Professor of Surgery, The Angeles Clinic and Research Institute, Cedars-Sinai Medical Center, Los Angeles, California

NORMA E. FARROW, MD
Department of Surgery, Duke University, Duke University Medical Center, Durham, North Carolina

ALEJANDRO R. GIMENEZ, MD
Division of Plastic Surgery, Baylor College of Medicine, Houston, Texas

ALICIA A. GINGRICH, MD
General Surgery Resident, Department of Surgery, University of California, Davis, Sacramento, California

BROCK B. HEWITT, MD, MPH, MS
Department of Surgery, Sidney Kimmel Medical College, Thomas Jefferson University, Philadelphia, Pennsylvania

GIORGOS C. KARAKOUSIS, MD
Department of Surgery, Hospital of the University of Pennsylvania, Philadelphia, Pennsylvania

AMANDA R. KIRANE, MD
Assistant Professor, Division of Surgical Oncology, Department of Surgery, University of California, Davis, Sacramento, California

RAGINI R. KUDCHADKAR, MD
Associate Professor, Department of Hematology and Oncology, Winship Cancer Institute, Atlanta, Georgia

KARENIA LANDA, MD
Department of Surgery, Duke University, Duke University Medical Center, Durham, North Carolina

MARGARET LEDDY, PA-C, MMSc
Department of Surgery, Duke University, Durham, North Carolina

ANN Y. LEE, MD, FACS
Assistant Professor, Department of Surgery, NYU Langone Health, New York, New York

MICHAEL C. LOWE, MD, MA, FACS
Assistant Professor of Surgery, Division of Surgical Oncology, Department of Surgery, Winship Cancer Institute of Emory University School of Medicine, Atlanta, Georgia

KELLY M. McMASTERS, MD, PhD
Ben A. Reid, Sr, M.D. Professor and Chair, The Hiram C. Polk Jr., MD, Department of Surgery, University of Louisville, Louisville, Kentucky

CONOR H. O'NEILL, MD
The Hiram C. Polk Jr., MD, Department of Surgery, University of Louisville, Louisville, Kentucky

DARRYL SCHUITEVOERDER, MBBS
Department of Surgery, The University of Chicago Medicine, Chicago, Illinois

ADRIENNE B. SHANNON, MD
Department of Surgery, Hospital of the University of Pennsylvania, Philadelphia, Pennsylvania

YUN SONG, MD
Department of Surgery, Hospital of the University of Pennsylvania, Philadelphia, Pennsylvania

JENNIFER TSENG, MD
Assistant Professor, Department of Surgery, The University of Chicago Medicine, Chicago, Illinois

CHARLES C. VINING, MD
Department of Surgery, The University of Chicago Medicine, Chicago, Illinois

SEBASTIAN J. WINOCOUR, MD, MS, FACS
Division of Plastic Surgery, Baylor College of Medicine, Houston, Texas

SANDRA L. WONG, MD, MS
Department of Surgery, Dartmouth-Hitchcock Medical Center, Lebanon, New Hampshire

XIAOWEI XU, MD
Department of Pathology and Laboratory Medicine, Hospital of the University of Pennsylvania, Philadelphia, Pennsylvania

Contents

An ambiguous pathologic report can present a clinical dilemma to the treating surgeon. We describe lesions ranging from the potentially benign to the likely malignant. Correctly identifying features associated with higher-risk lesions has proven challenging given the overall good prognosis and low rate of events. An appropriate treatment plan generally requires discussion between the surgeon and an experienced dermatopathologist. When clinically indicated, additional testing may be used to further support or refute a diagnosis of melanoma. The indications for these techniques, the data to support their use, and the strengths and weakness of each are reviewed.

Surgery with wide local excision is the mainstay of treatment for primary melanoma. Surgical margins differ depending on the depth of the primary lesion, subtype, and anatomic, cosmetic, or functional considerations. Adjuncts or alternative treatments to wide local excision are limited to specific patient populations and mainly experimental in nature.

Wounds resulting from wide local excision of melanoma vary in size and complexity, and require individualized solutions to achieve satisfactory closure. Goals of reconstruction include restoration of form, function, and aesthetics while minimizing donor site morbidity without compromising the effectiveness and safety of oncologic melanoma treatment. Optimal reconstruction relies on an in-depth understanding of the defect, locoregional anatomy and vasculature, available donor tissues, and basic wound healing and surgical principles. This article provides a broad overview of preoperative patient, timing, and wound considerations; various surgical techniques for complex reconstruction throughout the body; and postoperative care and complication management.

Age plays a dynamic role in incidence, presentation, and extent of disease for cutaneous melanoma. Even within the spectrum of juvenile melanoma, there exists a range of spitzoid and nonspitzoid melanocytic and melanoma lesions. Spitzoid melanomas, a more favorable disease in juvenile patients, are malignant lesions and require treatment as such. Lymph node metastases in melanoma occur at lower rates in older patients compared with younger counterparts, yet the rate of metastases is still high. Age appears to play an important role in the development and progression of melanoma, and understanding the differences across age populations is important when counseling patients.

Noncutaneous melanomas are rare subtypes of melanoma with high rates of metastatic disease and poor overall survival. One-third to one-half of cases are amelanotic, which may contribute to a delay in diagnosis. Immunohistochemistry staining with typical melanoma markers helps confirm the diagnosis. There is no standard staging system across mucosal melanomas. Elective nodal dissection is not recommended and there is a paucity of data to support use of sentinel lymph node biopsy. Mutational analysis should be routinely performed. Systemic therapy options include targeted inhibitors, immunotherapy, and cytotoxic chemotherapy, although further studies are needed to confirm their efficacy.

Sentinel lymph node biopsy is a key tool in the care of many patients with melanoma. The indications for the procedure have gradually become clearer over the 3 decades since the technique was developed. For appropriately selected patients, it carries enormous significance. Although it is a minimally invasive procedure, it does carry some risk. It is also a multidisciplinary procedure, requiring knowledge and experience from several specialties including nuclear medicine, surgery, and pathology.

Regional nodal melanoma management has changed substantially over the past 2 decades alongside advances in systemic therapy. Significant data from retrospective studies and from 2 randomized controlled trials show no survival benefit to completion lymph node dissection compared with observation in sentinel lymph node–positive melanoma patients. Observation is becoming the standard recommendation in these patients, whereas patients with clinically detected lymph nodes are still recommended to undergo lymph node dissection. Promising early results from a neoadjuvant approach inform the ongoing evolution of melanoma management. Recruiting patients to clinical trials is paramount to attaining evidence-based practice changes in melanoma.

Patients with unresectable cutaneous, subcutaneous, or nodal melanoma metastases are often candidates for injectable therapies, which are attractive for ease of intralesional delivery to superficial metastases and limited systemic toxicity profiles. Injectable or intralesional therapies can be part of multifaceted treatment strategies to kill tumor directly or to alter the tumor so as to make it more sensitive to systemic therapy. Talimogene laherparepvec is the only Food and Drug Administration–approved injectable therapy currently in wide clinical use in the United States, although ongoing trials are evaluating novel intralesional agents as well as combinations with systemic therapies, particularly checkpoint inhibitors.

With the universal adoption of immune checkpoint blockade and agents targeting BRAF-mutated melanomas in the metastatic setting, numerous clinical trials have evaluated these agents in the neoadjuvant setting. These smaller trials have shown promising results with high pathologic response rates and acceptable safety. Larger prospective randomized trials are under way to determine if all patients with resectable metastatic disease should be receiving neoadjuvant therapy.

This article presents the current data supporting adjuvant therapy for patients with cutaneous melanoma. With the recent development of novel immunotherapy agents as well as targeted therapy, there are strong data to support the use of these therapies in patients at high risk of developing recurrent or metastatic disease.

Clinical outcomes for metastatic melanoma have been dramatically altered by recent developments in immunotherapy and targeted strategies, but response to these therapies is not uniform, the majority of patients do not respond, and clinical response can be self-limited. Current directions in melanoma treatment aim to leverage a combination of therapies for tumors refractory to monoimmunotherapy, to include tumor-directed strategies, such as intralesional therapy and inhibitors designed for novel targets, which may augment current systemic agents when used in combination. Here, we summarize new classes of agents and emerging multimodal combination strategies that demonstrate significant promise in future melanoma management.

Stage IV melanoma has a 5-year survival rate of 6%, but considerable advances have been made in systemic therapies. Systemic immunotherapy has achieved durable responses in up to 40% of patients, with similar improvements with targeted therapies. This has reshaped the landscape for surgery in stage IV melanoma. Metastasectomy can be considered in patients on systemic immunotherapy or targeted therapy with responding, stable, or isolated progressing lesions, oligometastatic disease, or long disease-free intervals. Surgery plays a role in providing tumor tissue for preparation of tumor-infiltrating lymphocytes for adoptive cell therapy. Surgical palliation plays a role in patients with symptomatic metastases.

SURGICAL ONCOLOGY
CLINICS OF NORTH AMERICA

SERIES OF RELATED INTEREST

Surgical Clinics of North America
http://www.surgical.theclinics.com
Thoracic Surgery Clinics
http://www.thoracic.theclinics.com
Advances in Surgery
http://www.advancessurgery.com

THE CLINICS ARE AVAILABLE ONLINE!
Access your subscription at:
www.theclinics.com

Foreword

Management of Melanoma

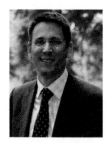

Timothy M. Pawlik, MD, MPH, MTS, PhD, FACS, FRACS (Hon.)
Consulting Editor

This issue of the *Surgical Oncology Clinics of North America* is devoted to covering the important topic of melanoma. The incidence of primary cutaneous melanoma continues to increase each year. While melanoma accounts for the majority of skin cancer–related deaths, surgical treatment of early disease can be curative. Over the last decade, there have been marked changes in the surgical and systemic treatment of melanoma. For example, within the surgical field, there have been multiple prospective randomized clinical trials to define the extent of surgery with important changes to how the nodal basin should be managed and staged. Among patients with advanced disease, treatment can be more challenging, although new advances in the area of immunotherapy now offer this group of patients more therapeutic options. In particular, the use of new laboratory, molecular, and imaging tests can better inform the initial workup of patients with newly diagnosed melanoma, as well as help tailor follow-up and personalized treatment options. As such, management of melanoma requires a well-informed multidisciplinary approach that incorporates surgeons, medical oncologists, among others, endocrinology, gastroenterology, medical oncology, and surgery. Surgeons therefore need to be well-informed about the emerging data on the diagnostic as well as surgical and systemic treatment options available for patients with melanoma.

I am thrilled to have Dr Keith Delman and Dr Michael Lowe guest edit this important issue of *Surgical Oncology Clinics of North America*. Dr Delman is the Carlos Professor of Surgical Anatomy and Technique in the Department of Surgery at Emory University School of Medicine, where he is Professor of Surgery and Associate Chair of Faculty and Clinical Affairs. Dr Delman is an international expert in the treatment of patients with melanoma. Dr Delman co-chairs the Winship Cancer Institute's Melanoma Working Group/Multi-Disciplinary Tumor Board at Emory, where he leads the multidisciplinary care of nearly half of all patients diagnosed with melanoma in the state of Georgia each year. Dr Lowe is an Assistant Professor in the Division of Surgical

Surg Oncol Clin N Am 29 (2020) xiii–xiv
https://doi.org/10.1016/j.soc.2020.03.003
1055-3207/20/© 2020 Published by Elsevier Inc.

Oncology of the Department of Surgery at Emory University School of Medicine. A board-certified surgeon, Dr Lowe serves as a surgical oncologist with a primary focus on cutaneous malignancy for the Division of Surgical Oncology within the Department of Surgery. He joined Emory after completing a fellowship in Complex General Surgical Oncology at Memorial Sloan Kettering Cancer Center in New York, New York. Given the combined knowledge and experience of Dr Delman and Dr Lowe, this duo of experts is ideally suited to be the guest editors of this important issue of the *Surgical Oncology Clinics of North America*.

The issue covers a number of important topics, including the workup as well as medical and surgical management of patients with melanoma. A wide array of expert authors reviews important surgical topics, such as operative margins, sentinel lymph node biopsy, management of the regional nodal basin, as well as reconstructive techniques. Other clinical locoregional and systemic topics, such as injectable therapies, neoadjuvant and adjuvant therapies, as well as novel targets and future therapies are covered. Furthermore, this issue addresses other topics, such as management of other age-related melanocytic lesions and noncutaneous melanomas. I want to thank Dr Delman and Dr Lowe for recruiting the help of such an amazing array of authors who are leaders in the field of melanoma treatment. Dr Delman, Dr Lowe, and all the authors do an expert job in summarizing the important and relevant aspects of caring for patients with melanoma. I would like to thank Dr Delman and Dr Lowe, as well as all the contributing authors for an excellent issue of the *Surgical Oncology Clinics of North America*.

Timothy M. Pawlik, MD, MPH, MTS, PhD, FACS, FRACS (Hon.)
Department of Surgery
Surgery, Oncology, Health Services
Management and Policy
The Ohio State University
Wexner Medical Center
395 West 12th Avenue
Suite 670
Columbus, OH 43210, USA

E-mail address:
tim.pawlik@osumc.edu

Preface

The (R)evolution of Melanoma Care

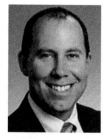
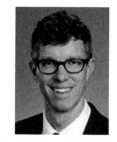

Keith A. Delman, MD, FACS   Michael C. Lowe, MD, MA, FACS
Editors

The management of melanoma has undergone a radical transformation over the past decade. Beginning with the publication of the Multicenter Selective Lymphadenectomy Trial-1 (MSLT-1) in 2006 and most recently with the results of the MSLT-2 trial in 2017, the surgical management of patients with this disease has evolved at a remarkable pace. In addition, substantial improvements in systemic therapy have prompted an exploration of neoadjuvant approaches, combination therapy, and many other attractive therapeutic endeavors. Technological improvements dating back to the 1990s have allowed modifications in approaches to regional therapy and even to surgical techniques. In addition, the evidence for novel agents, such as modified viruses and immune modulators, has grown and permitted a transformative change in our thinking about this disease. The future is full of possibilities and promise.

Regardless of what the future brings, it is critical that the surgical oncologist maintains a comprehensive understanding of the therapeutic landscape, both surgical and nonsurgical. A wise teacher once said that a surgical oncologist is really "an oncologist who uses surgery as their tool rather than systemic therapy or radiation." In that regard, surgical oncologists should be active leaders in the decision-making and care plans on the multidisciplinary team. Importantly, improvements in systemic therapy should encourage surgeons to reevaluate their role, rather than minimize or sideline it. The only cure for melanoma currently remains surgical extirpation. In many cases, treatment includes other components of multimodality care with which the surgical oncologist needs to be familiar. An in-depth understanding of the unique aspects of this disease, including considerations around age-related variation and pathologic interpretation, is therefore also critical to ensuring the surgeon is well equipped to provide input to the multidisciplinary team.

Surg Oncol Clin N Am 29 (2020) xv–xvi
https://doi.org/10.1016/j.soc.2020.03.002
1055-3207/20/© 2020 Published by Elsevier Inc.

surgonc.theclinics.com

It is our intent that this issue will provide the surgeon an overview that will help support their role in the increasingly complex care of the melanoma patient.

Keith A. Delman, MD, FACS
Division of Surgical Oncology
Department of Surgery
Winship Cancer Institute of Emory University School of Medicine
1365 Clifton Road NE
Atlanta, GA 30322, USA

Michael C. Lowe, MD, MA, FACS
Division of Surgical Oncology
Department of Surgery
Winship Cancer Institute of Emory University School of Medicine
1365 Clifton Road NE
Atlanta, GA 30322, USA

E-mail addresses:
kdelman@emory.edu (K.A. Delman)
mlowe3@emory.edu (M.C. Lowe)

Interpretation of the Complex Melanoma Pathology Report

Joseph G. Crompton, MD, PhD[a], Klaus J. Busam, MD[b],
Edmund K. Bartlett, MD[a],*

KEYWORDS

- Atypical melanocytic proliferations • Melanoma • Melanocytic nevus
- Molecular dermatopathology

KEY POINTS

- The varying classifications of ambiguous melanocytic lesions are reviewed.
- When pathologic ambiguity has significant clinical relevance, discussion between the surgeon and a dermatopathologist can guide the appropriate treatment.
- Additional testing, such as immunohistochemistry, comparative genomic hybridization, fluorescence in situ hybridization, and/or genetic analysis may aid in challenging cases.

INTRODUCTION

We have a sound understanding of the diagnosis, natural history, and treatment of both benign pigmented skin lesions and melanoma.[1-3] However, there are various pigmented skin lesions that bear a gross and histologic resemblance to melanoma or melanocytic nevi, but are neither clearly malignant nor benign. The incidence of these cutaneous lesions—collectively called atypical melanocytic proliferations—is not known, partly because a histopathologic diagnosis code does not yet exist to identify them. Although the incidence remains undetermined, these lesions are not uncommon in practice, provoking significant anxiety for patients and posing a substantial diagnostic and therapeutic challenge to surgeons.

First, the pathologist may struggle to find features of a lesion that can be reliably used to identify it. Some histologic characteristics (such as symmetric silhouette) may be consistent with a nevus, whereas other features (such as mitoses or atypia) within the same lesion are worrisome for melanoma. This leads to ambiguity in the

[a] Department of Surgery, Memorial Sloan-Kettering Cancer Center, 1275 York Avenue, New York, NY 10065, USA; [b] Department of Pathology, Memorial Sloan-Kettering Cancer Center, 1275 York Avenue, New York, NY 10065, USA
* Corresponding author.
E-mail address: bartlete@mskcc.org

Surg Oncol Clin N Am 29 (2020) 327–338
https://doi.org/10.1016/j.soc.2020.02.013
surgonc.theclinics.com

diagnosis and disagreement among pathologists when interpreting a biopsy specimen. Ultimately, some pathologists may merely report a diagnostic dilemma, not a diagnosis. Second, without a clear approach to identifying and characterizing these lesions, study of their natural history is highly problematic and indications for treatment remain uncertain.

The absence of a clear diagnosis, of course, does not relieve surgeons of the need to treat patients who come to clinic with an ambiguous pathology report. The therapeutic implications of our poor understanding of the natural history of atypical melanocytic proliferations is the possibility of overtreatment of lesions that pose no risk of harm and undertreatment of lesions that have real malignant potential. Here, we review the nomenclature, classification, and natural history of atypical pigmented cutaneous lesions to help the surgeon navigate the complex diagnostic and treatment approach required of these lesions. We focus our review on the basics of cytogenetic studies and mutational analyses that have clinical application for melanocytic tumors and discuss pitfalls in their interpretation.

NOMENCLATURE AND CLASSIFICATION

The nomenclature of various kinds of atypical melanocytic proliferations is as muddled as one might expect from a spectrum of pathologic entities that are poorly understood. Names frequently reflect the ambiguity: "minimal deviation melanoma," "borderline melanocytic tumor," "prognostically indeterminate melanocytic tumor," "atypical blue melanocytic neoplasms," "atypical Spitz tumor," "atypical spitzoid melanocytic tumor," and "atypical Spitz tumor of uncertain malignant potential."[4–9] The inconsistency and imprecision of diagnostic terms can vary between institutions, and imprecise descriptions do little to guide consistent and appropriate treatment.

To address this, there have been attempts to formalize ambiguous diagnostic terms for atypical melanocytic proliferations with the goal of standardizing reporting and simplifying treatment—the most notable 2 efforts being the World Health Organization classification of melanocytic tumors of the skin and the second being the Melanocytic Pathology Assessment Tool and Hierarchy for Diagnosis (MPATH-Dx). The MPATH-Dx includes 7 categories based on histologic criteria and consensus on therapeutic approach. Most of the atypical melanocytic proliferations are included in the "variable classification" group comprising class 2, class 3, and class 4. When applied by expert dermatopathologists the reported consensus ranges from 64% for class 2 lesions to 84% for class 3 lesions (50), highlighting the difficulty of reaching a consensus on diagnoses for lesions in the variable classification group.[10]

Until a more reliable classification system is developed and validated, a clinically relevant way to broadly classify the various terms describing melanocytic proliferations is simply whether the lesion is confined to the epidermis versus lesions with a dermal component. Lesions that are largely confined to the epidermis include atypical intraepidermal melanocytic proliferation (AIMP),[9,11–14] intraepidermal borderline melanocytic tumor (intraepidermal BMT),[13–21] and superficial atypical melanocytic proliferations of uncertain significance (SAMPUS).[22–26]

As discussed below, dermal lesions are associated with increased risk of melanoma, distant metastases, and melanoma-specific death. The grouping of melanocytic lesions that have a dermal component include dermal borderline melanocytic tumor (dermal BMT) and melanocytic tumors of uncertain malignant potential (MELTUMP)[22–26] (see **Table 1** for a summary of diagnostic terms).

Table 1
Diagnostic terms of atypical melanocytic proliferations

Diagnostic Term	Acronym	Description
Atypical intraepidermal melanocytic proliferation	AIMP	High-grade melanocytic dysplasia confined to epidermis
Superficial atypical melanocytic proliferations of uncertain significance	SAMPUS	High-grade melanocytic dysplasia confined to epidermis
De novo intraepidermal melanocytic dysplasia	DNIEMD	High-grade melanocytic dysplasia confined to epidermis, possible precursor to melanoma in situ
Pagetoid melanocytic proliferation	PMP	Atypical melanocytes (single or nested) throughout epidermis, including granular layer
Minimal deviation melanoma	MDM	Resembles acquired or Spitz nevi, but with vertical growth phase and has cellular atypia, such as melanoma
Intraepidermal borderline melanocytic tumor	Intraepidermal BMT	Atypical melanocytic lesion confined to epidermis
Dermal borderline melanocytic tumor	Dermal BMT	Atypical melanocytic lesion with thick dermal component
Atypical junctional melanocytic hyperplasia	AJMH	Melanocytes with more atypia than dysplastic nevi, but less than melanoma in situ
Melanocytic tumors of uncertain malignant potential	MELTUMP	Atypical melanocytes with thick dermal component

DIAGNOSIS AND INTERPRETATION OF THE PATHOLOGY REPORT

There are many things to consider when reading a pathology report to help inform treatment recommendations for cutaneous melanocytic proliferations. Because most diagnoses of melanocytic lesions are made by the morphologic evaluation of a biopsy specimen, the type and adequacy of the biopsy must be assessed. An adequate specimen must be taken to avoid sampling error, but there is an increasing trend toward smaller or more superficial biopsies. False-negative rates of melanoma initially diagnosed as melanoma in situ have been reported as high as 12% to 16%.[27,28]

Second, a pathology report of melanocytic lesions (that are not clearly melanoma) will not necessarily remark on Breslow depth or Clark's level, but the depth of the lesion—whether it involves the dermis or is limited to the epidermis—is important to note because it correlates with likelihood of distal or local recurrence.

Third, terms are occasionally used that are not pathologic diagnoses per se, but rather histologic descriptions when the diagnosis is uncertain. In this case, the pathologist is alerting the clinician to a diagnostic dilemma, not a diagnosis. This can happen, for example, when the pathologist is unable to exclude melanoma in situ because of the inadequacy of tissue or when there is no clinical knowledge of the lesion, such as size or appearance. There are also histologic features that can resemble melanocytic dysplasia concerning for melanoma in situ, but may arise because of inflammation or external trauma. One of the most common descriptors is AIMP. It is important for the surgeon to recognize when the pathologist is using a descriptive term, such as AIMP, because this may prompt the surgeon to either discuss the case further with the pathologist or ask for an opinion from another dermatopathologist. In the event that no consensus is reached and diagnostic uncertainly remains, there are ancillary diagnostic assays that may be requested to help clarify the diagnosis.

There are several assays that are in development to help shed light on the ambiguity of atypical melanocytic proliferations. Although staining with hematoxylin and eosin remains the gold standard in evaluating melanocytic lesions, emerging ancillary techniques are useful in cases of equivocal findings with conventional light microscopy. There are 4 categories of assays—immunohistochemistry, fluorescent in situ hybridization, cytogenetic studies, such as comparative genomic hybridization, and mutational analysis, such as gene expression assays—that are potential adjunctive tools to increase diagnostic accuracy (**Table 2**).

Immunohistochemistry

Basics
Immunohistochemistry is a microscopy-based technique and has been the primary adjunctive diagnostic tool to distinguish benign and malignant melanocytic tumors. The technique relies on labeled polyclonal or monoclonal antibodies that are specific for antigens of malignant cells not found on their benign counterparts.

Clinical applications
There are several immunohistochemical markers used in the evaluation of melanocytic lesions; S-100 remains the most sensitive marker for melanocytic lesions, but a handful of others, including MART-1/Melan-A, HMB-45, MITF, and tyrosinase have good specificity for malignancy. More recently, the melanoma-associated antigen PRAME (preferentially expressed antigen in melanoma) has been identified as both sensitive and specific for melanocytic tumors. In a study of 400 melanocytic tumors, diffuse nuclear immunoreactivity for PRAME was detected in 83% of primary melanomas and 87% of metastatic lesions. Of the 140 benign melanocytic nevi, 84% were completely negative for PRAME.[25–29] PRAME is emerging as a marker to distinguish malignant from benign melanocytic tumors.

Pitfalls
There are limitations with each of the melanoma-associated antigens used in immunohistochemistry to distinguish melanocytic tumors. Overestimation with Melan-A or underestimation with S100 of epidermal melanocytes can lead to overdiagnosis and underdiagnosis, respectively, of melanoma in situ.

Comparative Genomic Hybridization

Basics
The principal type of cytogenetic assay currently in use is comparative genomic hybridization (CGH), initially introduced in 1992, and more recently applied to melanoma. The goal of the technique is to evaluate for either gains or losses of either whole chromosomes or regions of chromosomes.[20,21] Total genomic DNA is isolated from both normal tissue and the tumor and labeled with various fluorochromes. The mixture is

Table 2
Molecular studies for diagnosis of atypical melanocytic proliferations

	Utility in Diagnoses	Advantage	Limitations
IHC	MIS; solar lentigines; and AIMP	Useful with limited tissue	Overestimation (with Melan-A) or underestimation (with S100) of epidermal melanocytes can lead to over- and underdiagnosis, respectively, of MIS
CGH	Benign melanocytic nevi and malignant melanoma	Evaluates full set of chromosomes	Not useful with limited and heterogeneous tissue
FISH	Melanoma, atypical melanocytic nevi, and ambiguous melanocytic proliferations	Optimal assay for limited amounts of tissue Sensitivity of 80%–100% and specificity of 95% for diagnosing melanoma	Targets only specific chromosomal aberrations False-positive tests secondary to polyploidy
Gene expression signature and mutational analyses	Benign melanocytic nevi and malignant melanoma	Classifies melanocytic lesions as benign or malignant with a sensitivity of 90% and a specificity of 91%	Further validation needed, especially in large cohorts of difficult atypical melanocytic proliferations and melanoma subtypes

Abbreviations: AIMP, atypical intraepidermal melanocytic proliferation; CGH, comparative genomic hybridization; FISH, fluorescent in situ hybridization; H&E, hematoxylin and eosin; IHC, immunohistochemistry; Melan-A, melanoma antigen recognized by T cells 1; MIS, melanoma in situ.

hybridized with metaphase chromosomes from a healthy donor (classic CGH) or genomic DNA (array CGH). Copy-number gains or losses are detected based on differences in fluorescence intensity.

Clinical applications
CGH is the most widely used diagnostic tool for the work-up of histologically ambiguous melanocytic proliferations. The most common chromosomal aberrations that distinguish melanocytic nevi from melanoma are gains in chromosome 7 with loss of 9q and 10.[30–32] The approach has an estimated sensitivity and specificity of 80% and 90%, respectively, but false-negative results may arise because of the failure to detect chromosomal aberrations in small populations of tumor cells (**Fig. 1**).

Pitfalls
Detection of an isolated copy-number change must be interpreted with caution. A Spitz nevus or tumor, for example, that show a loss of chromosome 3 or a gain in 11p, but otherwise lack worrisome features on morphologic analysis, are likely an indolent lesion. Heterogeneity in the tumor can also be a problem for interpretation

A

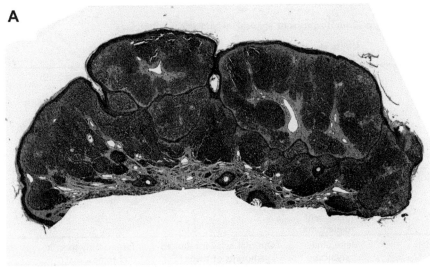

B

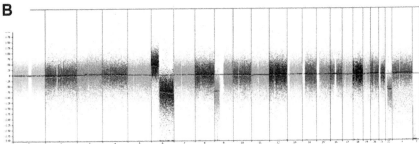

Fig. 1. Nevoid melanoma from the cheek of a young woman. (*A*) The microscopic findings of the lesion suggest a possible congenital nevus, but also showed features worrisome for melanoma. (*B*) SNP array analysis of the tumor revealed multiple unbalanced genomic aberrations, including gain of 6p, loss of 6q, and loss of 9p, including homozygous deletion of the CDKN2A gene, and loss of 22q.

of CGH. In general, roughly one-third of the tumor has to have copy-number changes to be detected by CGH.[33]

Fluorescence In Situ Hybridization

Basics

Fluorescence in situ hybridization (FISH) is an assay that evaluates individual chromosomes or particular regions within a chromosome. The basic technique involves binding of a fluorescently labeled oligonucleotide probe, specific for its complementary DNA sequence, and visualization with fluorescence microscopy. There are 2 general types of FISH probes—centromeric probes and allele-specific probes—relevant for the diagnostic work-up of atypical melanocytic lesions[33]. Centromeric probes bind to a centromeric region of a specific chromosome, thereby determining the number of copies of that chromosome. Allele-specific probes bind to a specific sequence of DNA to evaluate for aberrations that may be relevant to melanocytic lesions. One advantage of FISH is the ability to detect subpopulations of cells within a heterogeneous biopsy sample (**Fig. 2**).

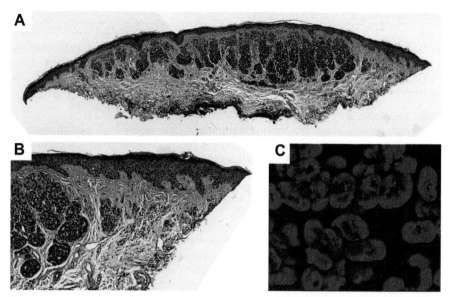

Fig. 2. Atypical melanocytic proliferation from the ear of an elderly man. (*A*) The patholo-gist who initially reviewed the findings was unsure as to whether the lesion was an atypical nevus or melanoma. (*B*) Juxtaposition of more densely cellular melanocytes with hyperchro-matic nuclei and adjacent blander nevus-like melanocytes at the edge of the biopsy. (*C*) FISH analysis revealed gains of 6p25 in more than 90% of atypical melanocytes, but not in the bland nevus cells. More than half of the atypical melanocytes also showed gain of 11q13 (not shown). A diagnosis of melanoma associated with a nevus was rendered.

Clinical applications

Compared with CGH, FISH can be more reliably used on biopsy specimens with limited tissue. It is also cheaper and more widely available because it requires less technical expertise. The 4-probe FISH assay—targeting genes on 6p25, 6q23, 11q13, and centromere 6—is used to differentiate between melanoma and benign nevi. The initial assay used to describe this approach had 87% sensitivity and 95% specificity for melanoma.[33] For diagnostically ambiguous melanocytic prolifer-ations, the use of FISH is mixed. In 1 study, Gerami and colleagues[34] examined 27 ambiguous lesions with FISH; all FISH-positive lesions ultimately metastasized.[16] Another study showed a specificity of 50% and a sensitivity of 60% for metastases.[23,35]

Pitfalls

There are several limitations to FISH. First, it only evaluates for genetic aberrations in the targeted areas, which is typically limited to 4 chromosomal loci. This is in contrast to CGH, which evaluates the complete set of chromosomes. Second, a negative FISH does not exclude malignancy. There are bona fide cases of melanoma diagnosed un-equivocally by morphologic studies that do not have copy-number changes on FISH. The specificity of FISH for melanoma is also not perfect. The most common scenario in which one sees false-positive FISH results arise is when benign lesions exhibit poly-ploidy. It has been shown that a minority of Spitz nevi, for example, is tetraploid in which there are 4 copies per nucleus of any chromosome tested. In this case, this is not a limitation of FISH per se, but rather the recognition that a gain in chromosomal copy number can be seen in unequivocally benign lesions.

Mutational Analyses and Gene Expression Signatures

Basics

A better understanding of melanoma genomics has enabled the use of mutational analyses as diagnostic adjuncts. Several genomic and somatic mutations in genes have been identified in melanoma, including PTEN, GNAQ/GNA11, KIT, MAP2K1/2, BRAF, and NRAS; many of these can also be detected in melanocytic nevi.[33]

Clinical applications

Mutational analyses show promise in discriminating melanoma from benign counterparts. In a study of 437 specimens, a 23-gene probe demonstrated a sensitivity of 90% and specificity of 91% in differentiating benign nevi from melanoma.[36] When this technique was compared with CGH, the results were largely similar in distinguishing melanoma and benign lesions, but showed discordant results for histologically ambiguous melanocytic proliferations.[37]

Pitfalls

Molecular studies have a lot of potential to help in the diagnosis of atypical melanocytic lesions for which conventional histologic techniques have reached their limits. Although all of these approaches require additional validation studies and long-term follow-up, each have utility, especially when ambiguity of diagnosis leaves us without one.

NATURAL HISTORY

The natural history of atypical cutaneous lesions, particularly the issue of whether they may progress to invasive malignancy, is poorly understood. There are a handful of observational studies that provide some insight. Here we will highlight studies of patients with a diagnosis of AIMP, DNIEMD, AJMH, MELTUMP, or dermal BMT on initial biopsy that was changed to melanoma or melanoma in situ after complete excision of the lesion. This does not necessarily provide a full understanding of the natural history of a lesion, but gives a sense of either the risk of misdiagnosing melanoma or the risk that a lesion may progress to melanoma after excision.

Regarding AIMPs, in an analysis of 306 patients with an initial diagnosis of AIMPs on biopsy, the final pathology of the surgically excised specimen changed to melanoma in 4.2% of patients (13/306).[11] Among these melanomas, most were melanoma in situ (11/13 patients, 85%), but 2 patients had invasive melanoma (2/13 patients, 15%). Risk factors associated with a change in diagnosis to melanoma included extension of the AIMP to the base of the biopsy specimen and location of the tumor on head, neck, and acral areas.

In a retrospective analysis of 82 skin biopsies initially diagnosed as DNIEMD, 8 lesions (9.8%) were melanoma.[38] This was consistent with a larger study of 263 patients with DNIEMD that described an increased association with dysplastic nevi and melanoma[39], suggesting that DMIEMD may be a precursor lesion or marker of increased risk of melanoma.

The likelihood of upstaging to melanoma from an initial diagnosis of AJMH was reported to be zero in a small retrospective study of 27 patients treated at a private dermatology practice.[40] Of the 27 patients, none were found to have melanoma on final surgical specimen. In addition, analysis of 19 patients (19/27, 70%) who had follow-up ranging from 2 to 6 years did not have recurrence of AJMH.

The risk of metastatic spread is thought to be higher for lesions that involve the dermis, such as MELTUMP and BMT. A prospective study of 32 patients with BMT who underwent both wide local excision and sentinel lymph node biopsy showed that the dermal variant of this lesion demonstrates regional lymph node involvement.[15]

Retrospective studies of MELTUMP showed lymphatic invasion in 25% of patients and this was associated with melanoma metastases and melanoma-specific death.[8] A retrospective review of MELTUMP tumors estimates the risk of developing regional metastases or disease-specific death from 1% to 2.4%.[41,42] Having noted this, it is important to emphasize that the natural history of lymph node involvement associated with MELTUMPS is far from clear. Regional lymph node involvement is not synonymous with malignancy; there are reports of bona fide benign nevi that spread to cutaneous lymphatics or lymph nodes.[23] Indeed, many MELTUMPs with involvement of lymph nodes demonstrated an indolent course.

Management

Although there are no evidence-based guidelines on treatment of atypical melanocytic proliferations, the general consensus is to stratify risk based on the layer of skin involved. For lesions confined to the epidermis on biopsy, surgical treatment is re-excision of biopsy site with negative margins. For atypical lesions involving the dermis, treatment involves wide local excision (ie, the same as melanoma) because of the afore-mentioned risk of distant metastases. Among the lesions with the dermal component, the most commonly reported are dermal BMT and MELTUMP.

A general principle of treatment of ambiguous cutaneous pigmented lesions is that the therapy should be adequate for the highest-risk entity in the differential diagnosis. If melanoma in situ or invasive melanoma is among the differential diagnosis, it ought to be treated as such. A second treatment principle is that clinicians must to be transparent in discussing the ambiguity of the pathology report and the difficulty of assessing the risk of frank malignancy. A discussion of whether to monitor, rebiopsy, or excise depends on factors that are not exclusively found in the pathology report. Adequacy of margins, for example, may differ based on anatomic location and the cosmetic results. A child with a completely excised conventional Spitz nevus on the eyelid, for example, may not warrant re-excision that results in a disfiguring scar, particularly if there is no diagnostic uncertainty or atypia.

There are alternative treatments for atypical melanocytic proliferations. Mohs micrographic surgery or staged excision can be considered for cosmetically challenging areas where adequate margins are difficult to obtain without disfiguring results. In patients who are poor surgical candidates, or with lesions such as lentigo maligna on the face that have expansive indeterminate boundaries, topical 5% imiquimod cream has been studied as an adjuvant treatment. One retrospective cohort study found that 94% of patients had clearance of lentigo maligna after treatment with surgery and imiquimod, with a mean follow-up of 43 months.[43]

SUMMARY

Here, we have highlighted the challenge of interpreting a pathology report that includes one of the many variants of ambiguous pigmented skin lesions. There are no consensus guidelines on treatment because fundamental questions about the nomenclature, classification, diagnostic criteria, and natural history of these lesions is poorly understood. Despite this poor understanding, surgeons must make real decisions in the clinic about whether to treat patients, knowing that the benefit of excising an atypical melanocytic lesion is unclear in many cases and potentially disfiguring. The reality of uncertainty demands that surgeons have as extensive an understanding as possible to help communicate to their patients the ambiguous nature of an atypical melanocytic lesion and its treatment.

DISCLOSURE

The authors have nothing to disclose.

REFERENCES

1. Kim JC, Murphy GF. Dysplastic melanocytic nevi and prognostically indeterminate nevomelanomatoid proliferations. Clin Lab Med 2000;20:691–712.
2. Briggs JC. Melanoma precursor lesions and borderline melanomas. Histopathology 1985;9:1251–62.
3. Cheung WL, Smoller BR. Dermatopathology updates on melanocytic lesions. Dermatol Clin 2012;30:617–22.
4. Mills OL, Marzban S, Zager JS, et al. Sentinel node biopsy in atypical melanocytic neoplasms in childhood: a single institution experience in 24 patients. J Cutan Pathol 2012;39:331–6.
5. Wick MR, Patterson JW. Cutaneous melanocytic lesions: selected problem areas. Am J Clin Pathol 2005;124(Suppl):S52–83.
6. Rywlin AM. Intraepithelial melanocytic neoplasia (IMN) versus intraepithelial atypical melanocytic proliferation (IAMP). Am J Dermatopathol 1988;10:92–3.
7. Pie rard GE, Pie rard-Franchimont C, Delvenne P. Simulants of malignant melanoma. Oncol Rev 2015;9:278.
8. Abraham RM, Karakousis G, Acs G, et al. Lymphatic invasion predicts aggressive behavior in melanocytic tumors of uncertain malignant potential (MELTUMP). Am J Surg Pathol 2013;37:669–75.
9. Zhang J, Miller CJ, Sobanko JF, et al. Frequency of and factors associated with positive or equivocal margins in conventional excision of atypical intraepidermal melanocytic proliferations (AIMP): a single academic institution cross-sectional study. J Am Acad Dermatol 2016;75:688–95.
10. Lott JP, Elmore JG, Zhao GA, et al. Evaluation of the Melanocytic Pathology Assessment Tool and Hierarchy for Diagnosis (MPATH-Dx) classification scheme for diagnosis of cutaneous melanocytic neoplasms: results from the international melanoma pathology study group. J Am Acad Dermatol 2016;75:356–63.
11. Zhang J, Miller CJ, Sobanko JF, et al. Diagnostic change from atypical intraepidermal melanocytic proliferation to melanoma after conventional excision—a single academic institution cross- sectional study. Dermatol Surg 2016;42:1147–54.
12. Chisholm C, Greene JF. Progression from atypical/dysplastic intraepidermal proliferations and carcinoma in situ to invasive tumors: a pathway based on current knowledge. Am J Dermatopathol 2011;33:803–10.
13. Urso C, Giannini A, Bartolini M, et al. Histological analysis of intraepidermal proliferations of atypical melanocytes. Am J Dermatopathol 1990;12:150–5.
14. Rywlin AM. Malignant melanoma in situ, precancerous melanosis, or atypical intraepidermal melanocytic proliferation. Am J Dermatopathol 1984;6(Suppl):97–9.
15. Magro CM, Crowson AN, Mihm MC, et al. The dermal-based borderline melanocytic tumor: a categorical approach. J Am Acad Dermatol 2010;62:469–79.
16. Magro CM, Abraham RM, Guo R, et al. Deep penetrating nevus-like borderline tumors: a unique subset of ambiguous melanocytic tumors with malignant potential and normal cytogenetics. Eur J Dermatol 2014;24:594–602.
17. Zembowicz A, Scolyer RA. Nevus/melanocytoma/melanoma: an emerging paradigm for classification of melanocytic neoplasms? Arch Pathol Lab Med 2011;135:300–6.
18. Scolyer RA, Murali R, McCarthy SW, et al. Histologically ambiguous ("borderline") primary cutaneous melanocytic tumors: approaches to patient management

including the roles of molecular testing and sentinel lymph node biopsy. Arch Pathol Lab Med 2010;134:1770–7.

19. Margo CE, Roper DL, Hidayat AA. Borderline melanocytic tumor of the conjunctiva: diagnostic and therapeutic considerations. J Pediatr Ophthalmol Strabismus 1991;28:268–70.
20. Weedon D. Borderline melanocytic tumors. J Cutan Pathol 1985;12:266–70.
21. Brodell RT, Santa Cruz DJ. Borderline and atypical melanocytic lesions. Semin Diagn Pathol 1985;2:63–86.
22. Elder DE, Xu X. The approach to the patient with a difficult melanocytic lesion. Pathology 2004;36:428–34.
23. Mooi WJ. "Lentiginous melanoma": full-fledged melanoma or melanoma precursor? Adv Anat Pathol 2014;21:181–7.
24. Zembowicz A. A new perspective for the classification of melanocytic lesions. In: 4th Melanoma Pathology Symposium of the International Dermatologic Surgery Melanoma Pathology Working Group. Tampa, FL: John Wiley & Sons; 2011; p. 1012.
25. Pusiol T, Piscioli F, Speziali L, Zorzi MG, et al. Clinical features, dermoscopic patterns, and histological diagnostic model for melanocytic tumors of uncertain malignant potential (MELTUMP). Acta Dermatovenerol Croat 2015;23:185–94.
26. Pusiol T, Morichetti D, Piscioli F, Zorzi MG. Theory and practical application of superficial atypical melanocytic proliferations of uncertain significance (SAMPUS) and melanocytic tumours of uncertain malignant potential (MELTUMP) terminology: experience with second opinion consultation. Pathologica 2012;104:70–7.
27. Mö ller MG, Pappas-Politis E, Zager JS, et al. Surgical management of melanoma-in- situ using a staged marginal and central excision technique. Ann Surg Oncol 2009;16:1526–36.
28. Hazan C, Dusza SW, Delgado R, et al. Staged excision for lentigo maligna and lentigo maligna melanoma: a retrospective analysis of 117 cases. J Am Acad Dermatol 2008;58:142–8.
29. Lezcano C, Jungbluth AA, Nehal KS, et al. PRAME expression in melanocytic tumors. Am J Surg Pathol 2018;42(11):1455–65.
30. Bastian BC, LeBoit PE, Hamm H, et al. Chromosomal gains and losses in primary cutaneous melanomas detected by comparative genomic hybridization. Cancer Res 1998;58:2170–5.
31. Bastian BC, Kashani-Sabet M, Hamm H, et al. Gene amplifications characterize acral melanoma and permit the detection of occult tumor cells in the surrounding skin. Cancer Res 2000;60:1968–73.
32. Bastian BC, Olshen AB, LeBoit PE, et al. Classifying melanocytic tumors based on DNA copy number changes. Am J Pathol 2003;163:1765–70.
33. Ensslin CJ, Hibler BP, Lee EH, et al. Atypical melanocytic proliferations: a review of the literature. Dermatol Surg 2018;44:159–74.
34. Gerami P, Jewell SS, Morrison LE, et al. Fluorescence in situ hybridization (FISH) as an ancillary diagnostic tool in the diagnosis of melanoma. Am J Surg Pathol 2009;33:1146–56.
35. Warner TF, Seo IS, Bennett JE. Minimal deviation melanoma with epidermotropic metastases arising in a congenital nevus. Am J Surg Pathol 1980;4:175–83.
36. Clarke LE, Warf MB, Flake DD, et al. Clinical validation of a gene expression signature that differentiates benign nevi from malignant melanoma. J Cutan Pathol 2015;42:244–52.
37. Wang G, Wang M, Alomari A, et al. Comparison of genomic abnormalities and gene expression analysis in atypical, ambiguous and malignant melanocytic

lesions. In: United States and Canadian Academy of Pathology Annual Meeting. Seattle, WA. 2016; p. 137A.

38. Sachdeva M, Frambach GE, Crowson AN, et al. De novo intraepidermal epithelioid melanocytic dysplasia as a marker of the atypical mole phenotype—a clinical and pathological study of 75 patients. J Cutan Pathol 2005;32:622–8.

39. Jessup CJ, Cohen LM. De novo intraepidermal epithelioid melanocytic dysplasia: a review of 263 cases. J Cutan Pathol 2010;37:852–9.

40. El Tal AK, Mehregan D, Malick F, et al. Atypical junctional melanocytic hyperplasia: a study of its prognostic significance. J Am Acad Dermatol 2012;66:AB141.

41. Kaltoft B, Hainau B, Lock-Andersen J. Melanocytic tumour with unknown malignant potential—a Danish study of 67 patients. Melanoma Res 2015;25:64–7.

42. Green RJ, Taghizadeh R, Lewis CJ, et al. Melanocytic tumours of uncertain malignant potential (MELTUMPs)—a diagnostic and management dilemma. Eur J Plast Surg 2015;38:13–6.

43. Swetter SM, Chen FW, Kim DD, et al. Imiquimod 5% cream as primary or adjuvant therapy for melanoma in situ, lentigo maligna type. J Am Acad Dermatol 2015;72:1047–53.

Margins of Melanoma Excision and Modifications to Standards

Brock B. Hewitt, MD, MPH, MS[a], Emma Bradley, BS[a],
Adam C. Berger, MD[b],*

KEYWORDS

• Melanoma • Excision • Margins • Mohs

KEY POINTS

• Excision margins are based on measured clinical margins at the time of surgery and vary depending on the depth of the primary melanoma.
• Certain melanoma subtypes, locations, cosmetic, or functional considerations may require modifications to standard resection margins.
• Mohs microscopic surgery has shown high local control rates, but remains an experimental treatment modality.

INTRODUCTION

Wide local excision of the primary lesion continues to be the mainstay of treatment for primary cutaneous melanoma. However, the extent of the excision has changed significantly over time. Debate surrounding the adequacy of excision margins dates to the late nineteenth century when surgeons, noting the aggressive nature and poor prognosis of the disease, recommended radical excision margins.[1,2] Furthermore, some surgeons advocated for extensive lymph node dissection to be performed in continuity with wide local excision such that, "all that is, removed should be in one continuous strip as far as possible."[3] This approach was supported in a landmark 1907 article published in *The Lancet* by Dr William Handley where he proposed wide margins to include fascial lymphatic vessels.[4] Over the ensuing decades, surgical margins extended out to 5 cm and many times included radical amputation. Evidence supporting such radical excisions came from studies such as the one by Olsen,[5] which reported atypical melanocytes up to 5 cm away from the primary

[a] Department of Surgery, Sidney Kimmel Medical College, Thomas Jefferson University, 1025 Walnut Street, College 605, Philadelphia, PA 19107, USA; [b] Cancer Institute of New Jersey, 195 Little Albany Street, Room 3005, New Brunswick, NJ 08903, USA
* Corresponding author.
E-mail address: Adam.berger@rutgers.edu
Twitter: @brockhewitt8 (B.B.H.); @DrABerger (A.C.B.)

Surg Oncol Clin N Am 29 (2020) 339–347
https://doi.org/10.1016/j.soc.2020.02.002

melanoma. She advocated for very wide excision margins to decrease the risk of local recurrence.[5]

During the early and mid-twentieth century, significant variation existed in the prognosis of cutaneous melanoma; reliable primary lesion characteristics were lacking. The unpredictable nature of the disease was, in part, a driving factor behind the practice of radical excision. However, studies by Trapl, Clark, and Breslow in the late 1960s found that vertical growth, and more specifically the depth of tumor invasion and tumor thickness, was a better prognostic factor than tumor size as determined by lesion diameter.[6–9] This belief was reflected in the American Joint Committee on Caner first edition using the level of primary lesion invasion and the thickness of penetration as the 2 factors determining primary tumor classification.[10] During this time, opposition to radical excision grew as evidence began to demonstrate similar survival rates with more conservative resection margins in certain patient populations. In his 1970 study establishing tumor thickness as a significant prognostic factor, Breslow[9] argued that patients with lesions less than 0.76 mm may be spared the morbidity of a prophylactic lymph node dissection, a common practice at the time. In a follow-up study in 1977, Breslow and Macht[11] found zero recurrences in 62 patients with thin melanomas (<0.76 mm), regardless of resection margin. In this study, 32% of patients had resection margins of 1.0 cm or less. The prognostic value of the histologic criteria introduced by these authors led to further investigation into the safety of more conservative margins.

Balch and colleagues[12] found no local recurrences in patients with primary melanomas less than 0.76 mm thick regardless of skin margins excised. Margins varied from 0.5 cm to 5.0 cm and 30% were less than 3.0 cm. They proposed a 2-cm excision margin with primary closure in patients with lesions less than 0.76 mm. Furthermore, investigators from the Sydney Melanoma Unit reviewed 1839 patients with stage I melanoma after wide local excision and 5-year follow-up.[13] In patients with thin lesions (0.1–0.7 mm), local recurrence rates were 0.6% in patients with excision margins of 2 cm or greater and 1.9% in patients with more narrow resection margins. The authors concluded that narrow excision margins were just as adequate for local disease control as wide excision margins in patients with thinner lesions. Finally, another large retrospective analysis by Urist and coauthors[14] evaluated the influence of surgical margins and prognostic factors for local recurrence in 3445 patients. In a subgroup analysis of 1151 consecutive patients with melanomas less than 1 mm thick, the authors found only 1 recurrence over the study time period despite excision margins of 2 cm or less in 62% of patients.[14]

Over the ensuing decades, prospective, randomized trails supported the conclusions of these earlier retrospective studies regarding the safety of more conservative excision margins guided by primary tumor characteristics. In this article, we discuss the data establishing current recommendations for surgical margins in primary melanoma and the circumstances when excision margins may be modified.

MELANOMA EXCISION STANDARDS

Cutaneous melanoma incidence has increased worldwide. Histologic factors of the primary lesion, specifically Breslow thickness and the presence or absence of ulceration, as well as nodal status drive melanoma-specific survival and, subsequently, melanoma staging. In the eighth edition of the American Joint Committee on Cancer Melanoma Staging System, the T stage is determined by the Breslow thickness with slight modification based on the presence of ulceration. Similarly, current standards regarding surgical excision margins are guided by the thickness of the primary lesion. In patients with resectable melanoma, current best practice guidelines support wide local excision of the primary lesion down to but not including the underlying fascia, with horizontal excision margins extending from the edge of the lesion, or biopsy site, up to, but not exceeding, 2 cm depending on the thickness of the primary lesion as permitted by anatomic, functional, or cosmetic considerations. Although certainly not settled, the recommendations are guided by multiple prospective randomized trials with long-term follow-up (**Table 1**).

The first published prospective randomized trial examining excision margins in primary melanoma was conducted by the World Health Organization Melanoma Program and began accrual in 1980.[15] In this multinational trial, 612 patients with primary melanoma no thicker than 2 mm were randomized to receive excision margins of either 1 cm or at least 3 cm. Disease-free and overall survival rates at 55 months were similar between the 2 study groups. Three patients had a local recurrence, all in the narrow margin group and all with a primary melanoma thickness of 1.0 mm or more. No local recurrences occurred in the wide excision group. In 1991, the authors published an updated analysis with a mean follow-up period of 90 months and found similar disease-free and overall survival rates.[16] The authors concluded, based on the absence of local recurrence in patients with a primary melanoma less than 1.0 mm and the very low rate of local recurrence overall, that 1-cm narrow margins are safe in patients with primary lesions no thicker than 2 mm.

Two prospective trials in Europe also examined patients with primary melanoma no thicker than 2 mm, but randomized patients to receive either 2 cm or 5 cm surgical margins.[17,18] First, the French Group of Research on Malignant Melanoma enrolled 337 patients from 9 European centers with a median follow-up time of 192 months. Local disease recurrence occurred in 4 patients who had a wide excision and 1 patient with a narrow excision. All local recurrences occurred in patients with primary lesions greater than 0.94 mm thick. No difference was found in 10-year disease-free or overall survival rates between the 2 study groups. The authors reported that 2-cm surgical margins were sufficient in patients with primary lesions 2 mm or less.[17]

The second European study was performed by the Swedish Melanoma Study Group and included 769 patients with a primary melanoma thickness ranging from

Table 1						
Randomized trials evaluating surgical margins after wide local excision of melanoma						
Trial	Year	n	Follow-up (Years)	Thickness (mm)	Excision Margins Compared (cm)	Survival
World Health Organization[15,16]	1988/1991	612	4.6/8	≤2.0	1 vs ≥ 3	NS
France[17]	2003	326	16	≤2.0	2 vs 5	NS
Sweden[18,19]	1996/2000	769/989	5.8/11	>0.8–2.0	2 vs 5	NS
Intergroup[20,21]	1993/2001	468	6/10	1.0–4.0	2 vs 4	NS
Sweden[24]	2011/2019	936	6.7/19.6	>2.0	2 vs 4	NS
UK[22,23]	2004/2016	900	5/8	≥2.0	1 vs 3	NSa

Abbreviation: NS, not significant.
a Analysis after median follow-up at 8.8 years showed a significant difference in melanoma-specific survival (unadjusted hazard ratio [HR], 1.24; 95% confidence interval [CI], 1.01–1.53; $P = .041$) favoring 3-cm margins but no difference in overall survival (unadjusted HR, 1.14; 95% CI, 0.96–1.36; $P = .14$).

0.8 mm to 2 mm. Seven local occurrences occurred, 3 in the narrow excision (2 cm) group and 4 in the wide excision (5 cm) group. No recurrences occurred in patients with a primary lesion thinner than 0.9 mm. Local and regional recurrence rates, as well as 5-year overall survival rates, were similar between study groups.[18] Long-term results from the Swedish Study Group included more patients (989) and a median follow-up period of 11 years. Local recurrence rates remained rare and no difference in survival was found between the study groups.[19]

The first randomized trial to investigate surgical margins in patients with intermediate thickness melanoma (1–4 mm) was conducted by Balch and colleagues.[20] They examined 486 patients, randomized to undergo surgical resection of either 2-cm or 4-cm margins. At a median follow-up time of 6 years, the rates of local recurrence and overall survival were not significantly different between study groups. The authors did find a significantly shorter length of stay in the 2 cm excision group, driven by the decreased need for skin grafting. Long-term results, with a median follow-up time of 10 years, also found no difference in local recurrence or overall survival between study groups.[21] However, the group reported that the presence or absence of ulceration profoundly influenced local recurrence rates. Overall, the authors concluded that 2-cm excision margins were safe in patients with 1- to 4-mm-thick primary melanoma. Together, these studies suggest that, owing to the low recurrence rates in primary melanoma lesions less than 2 mm, more conservative margins of 1 to 2 cm provide similar oncologic outcomes without the additional morbidity. However, prospective randomized trials directly comparing the safety of 1-cm with 2-cm margins are lacking.

As the push to more conservative resection margins continued, additional prospective studies were needed to elucidate the role of conservative margins in patients with more locally advanced disease. The first prospective study to exclusively include patients with a primary melanoma lesion at least 2 mm thick came from a group with participating institutions predominantly in the United Kingdom.[22] Researchers randomized 900 patients to receive a surgical margin of 1 cm or 3 cm. With a median follow-up time of 60 months, a 1-cm surgical margin was associated with an increase in locoregional recurrence (hazard ratio, 1.26; 95% confidence interval, 1.00–1.59; $P = .05$). However, there was no significant difference in melanoma-specific survival or overall survival between the 2 excision groups. Long-term data published by this group demonstrated lower melanoma-specific survival for patients in the 1-cm margin group (unadjusted hazard ratio, 1.24; 95% confidence interval, 1.01–1.53; $P = .041$), but the difference in overall survival was not significant.[23] The authors did note that surgical complications were nearly double in the 3-cm group (8% vs 15%). Overall, the authors suggested that 1 cm margins were inadequate for cutaneous melanoma thicker than 2 mm.

A second study examining patients with a primary melanoma lesion thicker than 2 mm randomized 936 patients over a 12-year period to undergo surgical resection with either a 2-cm or 4-cm margin.[24] After a median follow-up of 6.7 years, the melanoma-specific survival and overall survival were not significantly different between the 2 resection groups. Long-term data with a median follow-up period of 19.6 years confirmed the findings of the earlier study. The authors reported that 2-cm excision margins in patients with primary melanoma thicker than 2 mm was safe.

The final randomized trial worth discussing is the MelMarT trial published in 2018. In this feasibility study, 400 patients with stage T2 to T4 melanomas were randomized between and 1-cm and a 2-cm margin. This trial was not powered to examine local recurrence rates. However, the authors observed that there was a significantly higher rate of reconstruction in the 2 cm margin group (35% vs 14%; $P<.0001$), and the wound necrosis rate in the 2-cm margin cohort was significantly increased

(3.6% vs 0.5%; P = .036). Additionally, there was no difference in quality of life between the 2 groups at 12 months follow-up.[25]

A Cochrane review as well as a systematic review and meta-analysis have been performed of these randomized trials.[26,27] Although there are concerns over study heterogeneity, several conclusions can be drawn (**Table 2**). First, excision margins greater than 2 cm should generally be avoided.[26] Additionally, there are more data to support a 2-cm margin than a 1-cm margin for melanomas more than 1 mm thick, but no randomized studies have ever been done to perform a head-to-head comparison.[26,27] Across Europe and in the United States, general surgical excision margins are 1 cm for primary melanoma less than 1 mm thick and 2 cm for lesions thicker than 2 mm. For patients with melanoma between 1 and 2 mm thick, there is considerable variability in practice with surgeons choosing between a 1-cm and a 2-cm excision margin depending on prognostic characteristics and location. Several questions remain regarding appropriate surgical margins. Currently accruing patients is a phase III, multicenter, randomized controlled trail sponsored by Melanoma and Skin Cancer Trials, the national cooperative trials group of Australia and New Zealand, which is investigating 1-cm versus 2-cm surgical margins in patients with stage II (thickness >2 mm or 1- to 2-mm thick lesions with ulceration) primary melanoma (NCT03860883). Hopefully this study, a follow-up to the MelMarT study, will provide clarity for appropriate surgical margins in patients with thicker primary lesions and lesions with aggressive histologic features.

MODIFICATION TO EXCISION STANDARDS

Wide local excision with appropriate margins is the standard treatment for primary melanoma that is surgically resectable; however, owing to anatomic, functional, or subtype considerations, modification to the standard margins may be necessary. Unfortunately, a paucity of prospective data exists to guide appropriate melanoma resection margins in sensitive areas such as the face or distal extremities. Owing to functional or cosmetic considerations, even 1-cm margins may be difficult to obtain in these locations. Furthermore, there is debate surrounding the appropriate surgical margins in certain melanoma subtypes, as well as melanoma in situ.

Melanoma in situ, defined as cutaneous melanoma confined to the epidermis, and the most common subtype, lentigo maligna, present treatment challenges owing to the tendency to have ill-defined clinical margins in addition to the often, and yet unpredictable, subclinical extension of atypical melanocytes, potentially several centimeters beyond the clinical margins.[28] In patients with contraindications to surgical resection or significant cosmetic concerns owing to tumor location, alternatives include topical therapies (eg, imiquimod) or radiation. There is a lack of high-quality evidence

Table 2		
Recommended excision margins in primary melanoma		
Breslow Thickness	T Stage	Excision Margin (cm)
Melanoma in situ	Tis	0.5–1.0
≤1.0 mm	T1	1.0
>1.0–2.0 mm	T2	1.0–2.0
>2.0–4.0 mm	T3	2.0
>4.0 mm	T4	2.0

comparing nonsurgical and surgical treatment, but high histologic clearance and low recurrence rates have been achieved in experimental settings with experienced providers and close follow-up.[29–31]

Topical imiquimod has emerged as a therapeutic option as a neoadjuvant, adjuvant, or monotherapy treatment modality, especially in patients with lentigo maligna. In a retrospective review, Donigan and colleagues[32] reported a 3.9% recurrence rate at a mean time of 4.3 years in 334 patients with lentigo maligna who received imiquimod followed by planned surgical excision (median final margin of 2 mm). Swetter and co-authors[33] administered imiquimod as primary therapy (n = 22) or adjuvant therapy (n = 36) in patients with narrowly excised or histologically positive margins in the setting of lentigo maligna. At a mean follow-up period of 42 months, 16 patients (72.7%) in the primary therapy group and 34 patients (94.4%) in the adjuvant group demonstrated clinical clearance.[33] A literature review including 349 patients with lentigo maligna who received primary radiation therapy reported 18 recurrences (5%) over a median follow-up of 3 years.[31] Five patients had disease progression to lentigo maligna melanoma. Further studies are needed to clarify the role of nonsurgical treatments for melanoma in situ; however, current data suggest that reliance on topical or radiation therapies alone may put the patient at increased risk for local recurrence.

Historical guidelines recommended wide excision with 5-mm margins in patients with melanoma in situ; however, evidence suggests margins up to 1 cm are needed for adequate disease clearance, especially in lentigo maligna. A prospective cohort study of 2335 patients with melanoma in situ demonstrated clearance rates of 79% for lentigo maligna and 83% for nonlentigo maligna melanoma in situ with 6-mm margins. To achieve a 97% clearance rate for all melanoma in situ subtypes, a 12-mm margin was required on the head and neck and a 9-mm margin on the trunk and extremities.[34] As a result, current National Comprehensive Cancer Network guidelines recommend 0.5- to 1.0-cm margins for all melanoma in situ.

A growing body of evidence supports the use of Mohs microscopic surgery (MMS) for melanoma in situ in certain patient populations such as those with lentigo maligna of the face. Nosrati and colleagues[35] examined 662 patients retrospectively with melanoma in situ comparing wide local excision to MMS. They found no difference in 5-year recurrence rates, overall survival, or melanoma-specific survival. Furthermore, the use of MMS has increased in recent years and was the treatment modality of choice in more than 3% of all Surveillance, Epidemiology, and End Results–documented melanoma excisions from 2003 to 2008.[36] Chin-Lenn and colleagues[37] conducted a retrospective review comparing MMS (60 patients) and wide local excision (91 patients) in 151 patients with invasive melanoma of the face. The 5-year recurrence and disease-specific survival rates were not significantly different between resection techniques. On multivariable analysis, Breslow thickness was the only consistent predictor of recurrence or disease-specific survival. Overall, data on MMS are limited to retrospective review; prospective randomized trials are needed to clarify the ability of MMS to achieve high clearance and low recurrence rates before this approach can be considered a standard treatment option.

Primary melanoma located on the distal extremities in subungual sites, as well as the palms and soles, also present challenges to appropriate wide excision. In a retrospective review of 46 patients with subungual melanoma, the level of amputation did not affect survival or the incidence of local recurrence.[38] As a result, conservative amputation of the affected digit at the most distal interphalangeal or metatarsophalangeal joint is appropriate. In patients with plantar or palmar melanoma, the deep fascia should be preserved. These wounds are rarely closed primarily and generally require skin grafting or more extensive soft tissue coverage.

Certain melanoma subtypes, owing to their aggressive nature, may require larger resection margins than similarly sized cutaneous lesions. For example, desmoplastic lesions more commonly occur on the head and neck, are more locally aggressive, and may surround or directly invade nerves.[39] A retrospective review of 242 patients with either pure or mixed desmoplastic melanoma found that pure desmoplastic melanoma excised with 1-cm margins had higher incidences of local recurrence and mortality.[40] The authors recommended 2-cm margins even for thin lesions. Occasionally, radiation therapy is used as an adjunct to wide local excision of desmoplastic melanoma. A recent review of the National Cancer Database demonstrated a significantly improved overall survival for patients with desmoplastic melanoma treated with wide local excision plus radiation therapy compared with excision alone in multivariate analysis and propensity matching.[41]

Primary mucosal melanoma is a rare subtype, generally presenting at a more advanced stage, and has a worse 5-year survival than cutaneous or ocular melanoma.[42] Owing to the poor prognosis of these melanomas, treatment is conservative, favoring local excision instead of radical resection (ie, local resection instead of abdominoperineal resection for rectal mucosal melanoma). Radiation therapy does not improve survival but may improve locoregional control.

SUMMARY

Multiple prospective, randomized trials have demonstrated that less radical excision margins of primary cutaneous melanoma are noninferior and provide similar local recurrence and overall survival compared with more radical excision margins when guided by tumor depth. However, additional clinical trials are needed to clarify excision margins in certain patient populations, including those with lesions of intermediate thickness, aggressive characteristics, or located in cosmetically or functionally sensitive areas. Finally, although alternatives to wide local excision of the primary lesion exist, these techniques are still experimental and additional studies are needed to fully evaluate the efficacy of these treatment modalities.

DISCLOSURE

A. Berger has served on the Speaker's Bureau for Cardinal Health (Lymphoseek) and on Advisory Board for Castle Biosciences, Inc.

REFERENCES

1. Coats J. On a case of multiple melanotic sarcoma, with remarks on the mode of growth and extension of such tumours. Glasgow Med J 1885;24(2):92–7.
2. Snow H. Melanotic cancerous disease. Lancet 1892;2:872–4.
3. Pringle JH. A method of operation in melanotic tumours of the skin. Edinb Med J 1908;23:496–9.
4. Handley WS. The pathology of melanotic growths in relation to their operative treatment. Lancet 1907;1:92–1003.
5. Olsen G. The malignant melanoma of the skin. new theories based on a study of 500 cases. Acta Chir Scand Suppl 1966;365:1–222.
6. Trapl J, Palecek L, Ebel J, et al. Origin and development of skin melanoblastoma on the basis of 300 cases. Acta Derm Venereol 1964;44:377–80.
7. Trapl J, Palecek L, Ebel J, et al. New classification of melanoma of the skin. Acta Derm Venereol 1966;46:443–6.

8. Clark WH, From L, Bernardino EA, et al. The histogenesis and biologic behavior of primary human malignant melanomas of the skin. Cancer Res 1969;29(3): 705–27.
9. Breslow A. Thickness, cross-sectional areas and depth of invasion in the prognosis of cutaneous melanoma. Ann Surg 1970;172(5):902–8.
10. Carr DT. The manual for the staging of cancer. Ann Intern Med 1977;87(4):491–2.
11. Breslow A, Macht SD. Optimal size of resection margin for thin cutaneous melanoma. Surg Gynecol Obstet 1977;145(5):691–2.
12. Balch CM, Soong SJ, Murad TM, et al. A multifactorial analysis of melanoma. II. prognostic factors in patients with stage I (localized) melanoma. Surgery 1979; 86(2):343–51.
13. Milton GW, Shaw HM, McCarthy WH. Resection margins for melanoma. Aust N Z J Surg 1985;55:225–6.
14. Urist MM, Balch CM, Soong S, et al. The influence of surgical margins and prognostic factors predicting the risk of local recurrence in 3445 patients with primary cutaneous melanoma. Cancer 1985;55(6):1398–402.
15. Veronesi U, Cascinelli N, Adamus J, et al. Thin stage I primary cutaneous malignant melanoma. comparison of excision with margins of 1 or 3 cm. N Engl J Med 1988;318(18):1159–62.
16. Veronesi U, Cascinelli N. Narrow excision (1-cm margin). A safe procedure for thin cutaneous melanoma. Arch Surg 1991;126(4):438–41.
17. Khayat D, Rixe O, Martin G, et al. Surgical margins in cutaneous melanoma (2 cm versus 5 cm for lesions measuring less than 2.1-mm thick). Cancer 2003;97(8): 1941–6.
18. Ringborg U, Andersson R, Eldh J, et al. Resection margins of 2 versus 5 cm for cutaneous malignant melanoma with a tumor thickness of 0.8 to 2.0 mm: randomized study by the Swedish Melanoma Study Group. Cancer 1996;77(9):1809–14.
19. Cohn-Cedermark G, Rutqvist LE, Andersson R, et al. Long term results of a randomized study by the Swedish Melanoma Study Group on 2-cm versus 5-cm resection margins for patients with cutaneous melanoma with a tumor thickness of 0.8-2.0 mm. Cancer 2000;89(7):1495–501.
20. Balch CM, Urist MM, Karakousis CP, et al. Efficacy of 2-cm surgical margins for intermediate-thickness melanomas (1 to 4 mm). results of a multi-institutional randomized surgical trial. Ann Surg 1993;218(3):26–9.
21. Balch CM, Soong SJ, Smith T, et al. Long-term results of a prospective surgical trial comparing 2 cm vs. 4 cm excision margins for 740 patients with 1-4 mm melanomas. Ann Surg Oncol 2001;8(2):101–8.
22. Thomas JM, Newton-Bishop J, A'Hern R, et al. Excision margins in high-risk malignant melanoma. N Engl J Med 2004;350(8):757–66.
23. Hayes AJ, Maynard L, Coombes G, et al. Wide versus narrow excision margins for high-risk, primary cutaneous melanomas: long-term follow-up of survival in a randomized trial. Lancet Oncol 2016;17(2):184–92.
24. Gillgren P, Drzewiecki KT, Niin M, et al. 2-cm versus 4-cm surgical excision margins for primary cutaneous melanoma thicker than 2 mm: a randomised, multicentre trial. Lancet 2011;378(9803):1635–42.
25. Moncrieff MD, Gyorki D, Saw R, et al. 1 versus 2-cm excision margins for pT2-pT4 primary cutaneous melanoma (MelMarT): a feasibility study. Ann Surg Oncol 2018;25(9):2541–9.
26. Haigh PI, DiFronzo LA, McCready DR. Optimal excision margins for primary cutaneous melanoma: a systematic review and meta-analysis. Can J Surg 2003;46(6): 419–26.

27. Sladden MJ, Balch C, Barzilai DA, et al. Surgical excision margins for primary cutaneous melanoma. Cochrane Database Syst Rev 2009;(4):CD004835.
28. Higgins HW, Lee KC, Galan A, et al. Melanoma in situ: part II. Histopathology, treatment, and clinical management. J Am Acad Dermatol 2015;73(2):193–203.
29. Read T, Noonan C, David M, et al. A systematic review of non-surgical treatments for lentigo maligna. J Eur Acad Dermatol Venereol 2016;30(5):748–53.
30. Kai AC, Richards T, Coleman A, et al. Five-year recurrence rate of lentigo maligna after treatment with imiquimod. Br J Dermatol 2016;174(1):165–8.
31. Fogarty GB, Hong A, Scolyer RA, et al. Radiotherapy for lentigo maligna: a literature review and recommendations for treatment. Br J Dermatol 2014; 170(1):52–8.
32. Donigan JM, Hyde MA, Goldgar DE, et al. Rate of recurrence of lentigo maligna treated with off-label neoadjuvant topical imiquimod, 5%, cream prior to conservatively staged excision. JAMA Dermatol 2018;154(8):885–9.
33. Swetter SM, Chen FW, Kim DD, et al. Imiquimod 5% cream as primary or adjuvant therapy for melanoma in situ, lentigo maligna type. J Am Acad Dermatol 2015; 72(6):1047–53.
34. Kunishige JH, Doan L, Brodland DG, et al. Comparison of surgical margins for lentigo maligna versus melanoma in situ. J Am Acad Dermatol 2019;81(1): 204–12.
35. Nosrati A, Berliner JG, Goel S, et al. Outcomes of melanoma in situ treated with Mohs micrographic surgery compared with wide local excision. JAMA Dermatol 2017;153(5):436–41.
36. Viola KV, Rezzadeh KS, Gonsalves L, et al. National utilization patterns of Mohs micrographic surgery for invasive melanoma and melanoma in situ. J Am Acad Dermatol 2015;72(6):1060–5.
37. Chin-Lenn L, Murynka T, McKinnon JG, et al. Comparison of outcomes for malignant melanoma of the face treated using Mohs micrographic surgery and wide local excision. Dermatol Surg 2013;39(11):1637–45.
38. Heaton KM, el-Naggar A, Ensign LG, et al. Surgical management and prognostic factors in patients with subungual melanoma. Ann Surg 1994;219(2):197–204.
39. Chen JY, Hruby G, Scolyer RA, et al. Desmoplastic neurotropic melanoma: a clinicopathologic analysis of 128 cases. Cancer 2008;113(10):2770–8.
40. Maurichi A, Miceli R, Camerini T, et al. Pure desmoplastic melanoma: a melanoma with distinctive clinical behavior. Ann Surg 2010;252(6):1052–7.
41. Abbott J, Buckley M, Taylor LA, et al. Histological immune response patterns in sentinel lymph nodes involved by metastatic melanoma and prognostic significance. J Cutan Pathol 2018;45(6):377–86.
42. Mihajlovic M, Vlajkovic S, Jovanovic P, et al. Primary mucosal melanomas: a comprehensive review. Int J Clin Exp Pathol 2012;5(8):739–53.

Reconstructive Techniques in Melanoma for the Surgical Oncologist

Alejandro R. Gimenez, MD[a], Sebastian J. Winocour, MD, MS[b],
Carrie K. Chu, MD, MS[c],*

KEYWORDS

- Flap • Graft • Melanoma • Skin cancer • Skin graft • Reconstruction • Cancer
- Oncology

KEY POINTS

- Goals of reconstruction include restoration of form, function, and aesthetics while minimizing donor site morbidity without compromising the effectiveness and safety of oncologic melanoma treatment.
- Reconstruction of defects associated with wide local excision for the treatment of melanoma should take into consideration patient variables; disease factors; and anticipated defect location, dimension, characteristics, and surroundings.
- Reconstructive options include primary closure, healing by secondary intention, skin grafts, random-pattern flaps, and/or axial-pattern pedicled or free flaps of locoregional or distant origins.
- Multidisciplinary collaboration between the ablative and reconstructive teams in the preoperative, intraoperative, and postoperative periods provides comprehensive and safe treatments for melanoma patients undergoing surgical treatment.

INTRODUCTION

As the standard of care for primary cutaneous melanoma, wide local excision minimizes the risk of locoregional recurrence by including margins with tissue harboring local micrometastases, genotypically abnormal cells, and disease-free tissue.[1] Current guidelines recommend 1-cm lateral margins for lesions with Breslow thickness less than 1 mm and 1- to 2-cm lateral margins for melanomas thicker than 1 mm.[2]

[a] Division of Plastic Surgery, Baylor College of Medicine, 6701 Fannin Street, Suite 610, Houston, TX 77030, USA; [b] Division of Plastic Surgery, Baylor College of Medicine, 1977 Butler Boulevard, Suite E6.100, Houston, TX 77030, USA; [c] Department of Plastic Surgery, The University of Texas M. D. Anderson Cancer Center, 1400 Pressler Street, Unit 1488, Houston, TX 77030, USA
* Corresponding author.
E-mail address: CKChu@mdanderson.org
Twitter: @AGimenezMD (A.R.G.); @WinocourMD (S.J.W.); @DrCarrieChu (C.K.C.)

Surg Oncol Clin N Am 29 (2020) 349–367
https://doi.org/10.1016/j.soc.2020.02.003
1055-3207/20/© 2020 Elsevier Inc. All rights reserved.

surgonc.theclinics.com

Deep margins should extend to, and sometimes include, the underlying deep fascia. Resultant defects may have significant functional and aesthetic implications, particularly in the head and neck and extremities. A multidisciplinary team with early involvement of a reconstructive surgeon allows for appropriate planning and execution, and ensures optimal results with low local recurrence rates.

Wounds resulting from wide local excision vary in size and complexity, and require individualized solutions to achieve functional and aesthetic closures. Optimal reconstruction relies on an in-depth understanding of the defect, locoregional anatomy and vasculature, available donor tissues, and basic wound healing and surgical principles and techniques. This article provides a broad overview of preoperative patient, timing, and wound considerations; various surgical techniques; and postoperative care and complication management.

PREOPERATIVE CONSIDERATIONS
Patient Factors

The success of reconstructive surgery depends on preoperative consideration and optimization of patient-related risk factors that should be elicited through a comprehensive history and examination. It is imperative to screen the patient for comorbidities that may complicate wound healing or preclude prolonged surgery, such as obesity, diabetes mellitus, chronic obstructive pulmonary disease, hypertension, cardiovascular or peripheral vascular disease, renal disease, coagulopathies, rheumatologic disorders, or immunocompromised and malnutrition states.[3,4] Medications, such as anticoagulants or steroids, may complicate the surgery or postoperative course.[5] Prior history of radiation at the site of surgery or tobacco use may decrease tissue vascularity and perfusion.[4,6] Actively smoking patients should be counseled on smoking cessation and, if timing allows, encouraged to discontinue smoking at least 4 weeks before surgery.[7] Age and preoperative functional and ambulatory capacity may inform the type of reconstruction a patient may be able to tolerate. Patient expectations, reconstructive options and their possible complications, and anticipated functional and cosmetic outcomes should be addressed preoperatively.

Reconstructive Timing

The optimal timing of reconstruction after melanoma excision remains a topic of debate. Although Mohs micrographic surgery is widely used in the excision of nonmelanoma cutaneous malignancies, frozen section analysis of melanoma has not been shown to be reliable or accurate enough for routine use.[8,9] Because negative margin status cannot be confirmed intraoperatively, surgeons have traditionally delayed reconstruction or limited immediate reconstruction to skin grafts while awaiting permanent pathology. Skin grafting facilitates continued ease of surveillance without distorting the local anatomy or masking recurrent disease. Although this traditional approach is safe oncologically, it inconveniences the patient, requires further anesthetic episodes, and increases health care costs.[10,11] Whenever possible, patients prefer a single procedure with immediate reconstruction to avoid a prolonged period of disfigurement.[12]

Although there are a small number of studies exploring the optimal timing of reconstruction, recently, immediate reconstruction following wide local excision of melanoma has been performed with safe and reassuring outcomes.[10,11,13] A recent systematic review by Quimby and colleagues[13] concluded similar rates of positive margins and local recurrence between delayed and immediate reconstruction. Furthermore, locally recurrent, ulcerated, thicker melanomas (T4), melanoma in situ with ill-defined borders, and desmoplastic melanomas have been identified as high-risk for positive margins; delayed reconstruction may be more prudent in these cases.[10,11] More complex reconstructions with adjacent tissue rearrangement and locoregional flaps have been shown to be safe because they often allow for larger excision margins and they do not impede re-excision in the case of positive margins.[6,10,11,13] More high-quality studies are needed to further define guidelines for reconstructive timing.

DEFECT ASSESSMENT

An optimal reconstruction provides adequate and safe coverage of a given defect, restores tissue composition, and preserves form and function while minimizing donor site morbidity. Reconstruction begins with thorough assessment of the wound, surrounding tissues, and a survey of available donor tissues. The location, size, depth, tissue quality, skin thickness and laxity, vascularity, and any lost or exposed underlying critical structures must all be described. Adjacent functional structures or organs should be noted to avoid their disruption. If delayed reconstruction is performed, viable, desiccated, and necrotic tissues must be differentiated, and any slough, eschar, or signs of infection must be addressed. Although these basic principles can guide general wound assessment, there are special considerations unique to each body part that inform the required reconstruction.

Head and Neck

The head and neck region is a particularly challenging area for reconstruction because the delicate aesthetic and functional demands are extensive. Minor reconstructive flaws are readily evident. Within the face, there are static and dynamic structures with several special function organs, including the orbit and its contents, nose, ears, lips, and mouth.[14,15] To guide wound assessment and reconstruction, facial anatomy is divided into various aesthetic subunits determined by skin quality, thickness, color, texture, contour, and function.[5,16,17] Delimiting the reconstruction by aesthetic subunits may yield superior results, because scars may be concealed at the boundaries between these topographic subunits. Favorable incision design allows for eventual scar camouflage within Langer lines of tension. One should aim to replace lost tissues with "like" counterparts that exhibit similar color and thickness. Given the density of critical anatomy in this region, specific potential complications should be discussed preemptively, and intraoperative measures should be undertaken to limit such morbidity. Preservation of facial nerve motor branch function is important during the ablative and reconstructive procedures. Forehead reconstructions should consider hairline disruption. Periocular reconstructions should avoid designs that may predispose to ectropion, especially in elderly patients with lower lid laxity at baseline.

Extremities

The upper extremity poses its own reconstructive challenges. As the upper extremity tapers in circumference from proximal to distal, skin laxity and donor tissues diminish and bones are located in a more superficial subcutaneous plane, making reconstructions more complex. The surgeon must consider the complex functionality and extensive range of motion of the numerous joints, avoiding any options that may limit motion or cause stiffness, because these can result in long-term disability. Durable coverage of vital structures, such as exposed muscles, tendons, vessels, and nerves, should also allow for muscle and tendon gliding while maintaining neurovascular integrity of the upper extremity.[17,18]

The lower extremity poses many of the same challenges, because it has diminishing amounts of skin laxity, subcutaneously positioned bones and vital structures, and high functionality with extensive range of motion. Additionally, the lower extremity is a weight-bearing structure that withstands significant pressure and shearing forces and requires intact sensory innervation. Wound reconstruction should be robust and durable. The sensory function of the plantar foot should be preserved. Even small wounds can result in bone exposure in the distal third of the leg, which may require reconstruction with free flaps. Underlying peripheral vascular disease should be recognized and optimized to enhance healing potential.[17,18]

Trunk

The chest, abdomen, and back are generally forgiving because there is ample tissue laxity amenable to primary closure. The groin, which harbors important neurovascular structures, does require durable and well-vascularized coverage that obliterates the existing dead space and minimizes the risk of infection and compromise of critical structures.[17]

SURGICAL TECHNIQUE

To help the reconstructive surgeon conceptualize all the surgical options in a systematic approach, Mathes and Nahai introduced the metaphor of the reconstructive ladder.[19] This concept allows the surgeon to consider various wound closure options in a stepwise fashion from the simplest to the most complex, tailoring each solution to a patient's specific reconstructive, health, and functional needs. Over the years, the ladder has been adapted to include newer modalities of wound care and closure and now includes: closure by secondary intention, direct primary closure, skin graft, dermal matrices, local flaps or tissue rearrangement, regional flaps, tissue expansion, and free flaps (**Fig. 1**).[20] Negative pressure wound therapy can serve as an adjunct to every

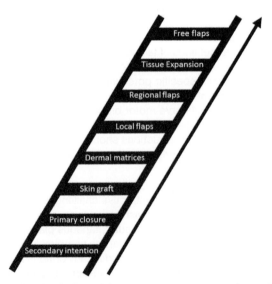

Fig. 1. Reconstructive ladder. (*Adapted from* Janis JE, Kwon RK, Attinger CE. The new reconstructive ladder: modifications to the traditional model. *Plastic and reconstructive surgery.* 2011;127 Suppl 1:205s-212s.)

possibility. The ladder should not be adhered to in a strict order where the best option is the simplest option. Rather, it should serve as a simple framework to consider all the available options and the final solution should be tailored to the patient.

Primary Closure and Secondary Intention Healing

Simple closures can generate favorable aesthetic and functional results. Primary closure outcomes may be optimized by placing incisions for ablative procedures along the boundaries of aesthetic subunits or along the relaxed skin tension lines. Linear closure over a joint surface should preserve sufficient laxity to accommodate full range of motion. Closure by secondary intention may be appropriate in locations where wound contraction would not cause undue morbidity, such as on the trunk, proximal extremities, or scalp. Wounds on facial concavities, such as on the inner canthus, alar crease, and within the helical rim, are known to heal successfully with good cosmetic and functional results. However, management requires regular wound care. The aesthetic outcomes are unpredictable and may require revisionary surgery.[21]

Skin Grafts

Skin grafts have been used traditionally to close melanoma defects because they allow for continued surveillance without anatomic distortion. By definition, grafts are tissues that are harvested from one part of the body, completely devascularized, and then replaced at the wound, where they survive via a three-stage process of imbibition, inosculation, and neo/revascularization. During the initial imbibition stage, which lasts about 24 to 48 hours, the graft, which is held in place by a thin and delicate fibrin layer, survives by diffusion of nutrients from the wound bed. Following this phase, the end capillaries from the recipient wound bed and graft begin to align in a process known as inosculation, and, over the course of several days, become mature arterial and venous vessels. The success of this process depends on the presence of a healthy, well-vascularized wound bed; prevention of seromas, hematomas, or infections; and minimizing shearing forces on the graft.[22]

Depending on the depth of harvest and the amount of dermis included, skin grafts are classified as split-thickness or full-thickness. Split-thickness skin grafts (STSG), which are harvested at a depth of 0.012 to 0.020 inches, contain varying amounts of dermis. By contrast, full-thickness skin grafts (FTSG) contain the entire dermis and are harvested down to the underlying subcutaneous tissue. The variable amount of dermis confers several important graft characteristics. First, FTSG exhibit greater degrees of primary contraction, because the elastin fibers within the dermis cause an immediate recoil following harvest. However, secondary contraction, which occurs in delayed fashion within a healed graft, is greater for an STSG. FTSG have the ability to regenerate sweat glands, grow hair, and become reinnervated because epithelial appendages and neurilemmal sheaths are transferred within the dermis. Finally, FTSG have an increased risk of failure or partial take, because their metabolic requirements are greater.[22]

The donor site for graft harvest may be chosen based on the color, texture, thickness, and size of graft required. STSG are harvested from the lateral thighs, buttocks, trunk, or even scalp. By contrast, FTSG are harvested from the groin, preauricular or postauricular regions, the supraclavicular regions, and the gluteal crease. FTSG sizing is limited by the capacity for primary donor site closure. Although a graft can be meshed to increase its size and allow for drainage of underlying fluids, it does result in a more unsightly result.[22]

Although skin grafts provide a technically simple and quick reconstructive option and allow for continued easy surveillance, there are several disadvantages. STSG donor sites are painful, heal by secondary intention, and are ultimately unsightly. Hypopigmentation or hyperpigmentation, texture and contour irregularities, and contracture may compromise recipient site appearance. Finally, in the long-term, skin grafts do not tolerate trauma or repetitive forces well and can break down easily, requiring further revisions. Although skin grafts are an indispensable technique for reconstruction, advances in surgical technique and evolving knowledge of flap anatomy and physiology may make these complex reconstructions more appealing solutions.[22]

Flaps

Flap surgery, whether from locoregional or distant tissues, provides a more sophisticated means of reconstruction with the aim of improving functional and aesthetic results and minimizing donor site morbidity. In contrast to grafts, flaps maintain their own blood supply and do not depend on the recipient wound bed vascularity for survival. Therefore, flaps can be used for defects with poorly vascularized or devascularized wound beds. Locoregional flaps are classified by their blood supply into random or axial pattern flaps.[23] Random-pattern flaps are supplied by the subdermal plexus, whereas axial pattern flaps are supplied by a specific named and identifiable cutaneous artery within the longitudinal axis of the flap. Traditionally, the dimensions of these flaps are limited to a length-to-width ratio of 2 to 3:1 for random pattern flaps to 6:1 for axial pattern flaps. As this ratio increases, the risk of flap necrosis increases.[24] When the locoregional tissues are not apt for defect closure, more extensive and larger pedicled or free flaps can be performed. In the following sections, several fundamental random- and axial-pattern flaps used to reconstruct defects throughout the body are described.

Random pattern flaps

Advancement flaps Advancement flaps recruit adjacent tissues to close the defect in a linear fashion. The skin edge moves unidirectionally forward without any rotation or lateral movement.[25] There are various iterations of the advancement flap. The single advancement flap is designed as a square or rectangular flap in which two parallel incisions are made along tangents to the wound edges. The flap is then elevated at a depth to match the contour of the defect. Flap advancement distance is increased by excising Burow triangles laterally at the base of the flap. If a single-pedicle advancement flap does not suffice, two opposing single-pedicle advancement flaps can be performed to provide additional tissue to achieve wound closure (**Fig. 2**).

The V-Y advancement flap is designed as a triangle with two divergent incisions from a point of origin to opposing edges of the wound (**Fig. 3**). The angle between these diverging lines should be about 30°, because this allows for the length of the triangle to be about two to three times larger than the defect diameter. The width of the triangle should be equal to the defect diameter.[25] The resultant triangular skin island must not be undermined to preserve vascularity. Instead, undermining of the wound edges and island flap perimeter should be performed to allow for tension-free closure. The final suture lines create a Y-shape.

The keystone flap has recently emerged as a novel and versatile solution that finds particular applicability in distal limbs.[26] The design and movement of this flap draws on the foundation of the more classic advancement flaps. Flap design begins with excision of a lesion within an ellipse along the longitudinal direction. The flap is then performed over the area of most tissue laxity. Two incisions are planned at proximal and distal ends of the defect at 90° angles to the wound edge. From these incision end

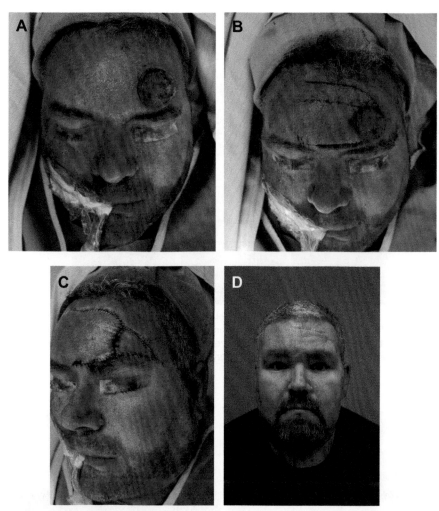

Fig. 2. Advancement flap. (*A*) Circular defect involving left forehead immediately adjacent to eyebrow. (*B*) Medially based forehead advancement flap. (*C*) Intraoperative flap inset and closure. Additional lateral V-Y advancement was performed for additional coverage. (*D*) Final results at 6 months.

points, a curvilinear arc parallel to the wound edge is designed to connect to these two end points. An islandized flap is created by making full-thickness incisions without beveling. Along the greater arc, a fasciotomy is performed to maximize mobility. The skin island should not be undermined. After dissection is completed, closure should begin at the proximal and distal edges in a V-Y fashion with the goal of providing enough tissue laxity centrally to close the defect (**Fig. 4**).[26]

Larger defects are amenable to closure with double keystone flaps. In the lower extremities, keystone flaps have allowed for fast recovery times, short time to ambulation, reduced postoperative pain, and improved cosmetic results with minimal donor site morbidity.[27] Furthermore, the flap allows for appropriate excision margins and does not complicate re-excision in the event of positive margins.

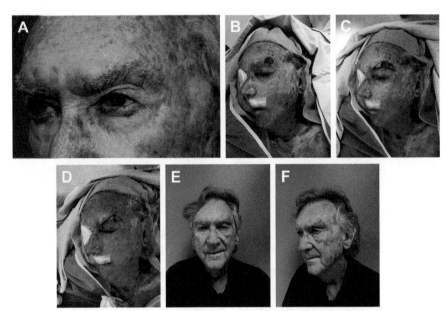

Fig. 3. V-Y advancement. (*A*) Preoperative melanoma involving the left eyebrow. (*B*) Left eyebrow defect following wide local excision of melanoma. (*C*) Double opposing V-Y advancement flaps designed along natural eyebrow curvature. (*D*) Intraoperative tension-free flap inset with viable flaps. (*E, F*) Postoperative results at 4 weeks.

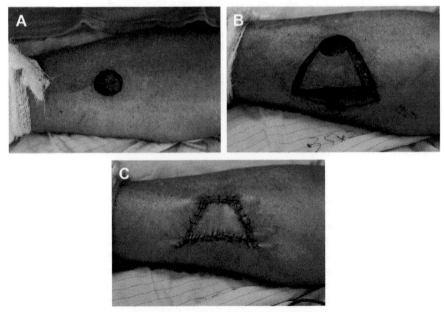

Fig. 4. Keystone flap. (*A*) Full-thickness circular defect involving the medial leg. (*B*) Keystone flap is incised down to the underlying fascia. (*C*) Intraoperative flap inset and closure with V-Y closure at proximal and distal edges.

Rotational flaps When defects cannot be closed along a single tension vector by primary closure or with advancement flaps, rotational flaps are used to turn a semicircular flap of lax adjacent skin and subcutaneous tissue about a pivot point. An arc is drawn extending from the base of the defect onto the adjacent lax tissues. The flap and its surrounding tissues should be widely undermined. When planning these flaps, the arc length, degree of curvature, and expected degree of rotation should inform flap design to ensure adequate wound coverage.[28,29] The effective length of a flap decreases as the degree of rotation about its pivot point increases. Thus, the arc length should be longer than the defect itself. To maximize movement, the optimal arc of rotation should be from 90° to 180°. If rotation is hindered at the pivot point, a back-cut extending into the base of the flap may be performed to allow for greater arc of rotation. The appropriate back-cut strikes a fine balance between flap mobility and vascular compromise. After the flap is rotated into place, a secondary donor site defect is created, which can usually be closed primarily or with a skin graft. This scenario most commonly occurs on the scalp, where flap coverage over denuded calvarium may be achieved while preserved pericranium at the donor defect is amenable to skin graft coverage (**Fig. 5**).

Rotational flaps are commonly used for large defects in the scalp, cheeks, and trunk. The cervicofacial rotational flap is a workhorse option for cheek defects within the suborbital and preauricular regions because it provides tissue with appropriate color, texture, contour, and hair match (**Fig. 6**). The flap may be based anteriorly or posteriorly. The variable extent of the incisions typically course along the nasolabial fold, the cheek-lid junction toward the outer canthus, the temple and temporal hairline, preauricular skin, and the retroauricular scalp or neck skin.[30] The incision extent depends on the exact defect location and dimensions. Widely versatile, this flap elegantly exploits the generous cutaneous lower face and neck laxity typically accumulated with age. However, the most distal aspect of the flap has a tenuous blood supply. In smokers, a deep-plane cervicofacial rotation advancement flap, which has a more robust blood supply because of inclusion of the platysma, may reduce the risk of partial flap necrosis.[31] Design should avoid downward tension vectors against the lower lid, which may result in ectropion. In at-risk patients, preemptive canthopexy may be prudent. Careful planning of any necessary cervical nodal dissection incisions with the ablative surgeon, especially in staged surgeries, preserves optimal cervicofacial flap incisional design. The skin flap may even be undermined and elevated in part by the reconstructive surgeon first to facilitate neck access.

The ying-yang flap is another rotational flap variant, consisting of two double opposing rotational flaps. The arcs are designed in opposing sides of a wound in either a clockwise or counterclockwise fashion, which allows for both flaps to be rotated in opposite directions into the defect. This closure technique is particularly helpful within the scalp, because the extensive vascular network can supply various rotational flaps and the patient's hair will conceal the incisions. Extensive undermining of the rotational flaps is required for closure because scalp tissue is inelastic, and tension-associated alopecia should be minimized.[5] The addition of multiple additional rotation flaps around a circular defect creates the "pin-wheel" flap.

Transposition flaps Transposition flaps are rectangular or square pedicled flaps that are recruited from adjacent tissues and rotated about a pivot point into a defect.[32] Many of the same principles that dictate rotational flap design also govern transposition flap planning. Typically smaller than rotational flaps, the donor sites can usually be closed primarily. There are numerous types of transposition flaps that are used throughout the body.

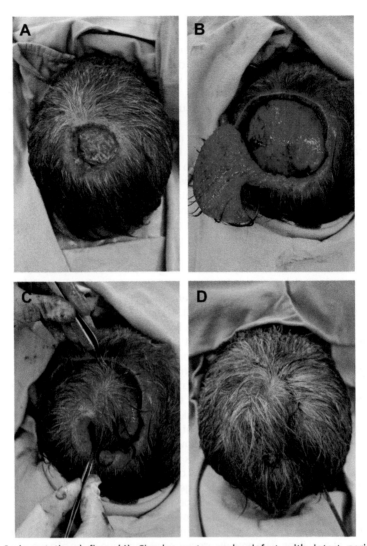

Fig. 5. Scalp rotational flap. (*A*) Circular vertex scalp defect with intact pericranium following excision of melanoma. (*B*) Adjacent rotational scalp flap elevated in a subgaleal plane with underlying pericranium intact. (*C*) Flap rotated into defect. (*D*) Intraoperative tension-free flap inset without distortion of hair direction.

The rhomboid flap was first described by Limberg.[33] The key initial step is to convert the defect into a rhombus, or a four-sided parallelogram with equal sides (x) and opposing 60° and 120° angles. From the vertex at one of the 120° angles, an outward incision of length x is made and, from this incision end point, a second incision parallel to the sides of the rhombus is made, forming a 60° angle (**Fig. 7**). Because there are four possible flap configurations for any rhomboid defect, the expected donor site should be placed over the site of maximal tissue laxity. Once the flap and donor sites are reapproximated, the resulting suture line should resemble a question mark. These versatile flaps are applied to defects throughout the body, but are especially popular in the trunk and extremities.

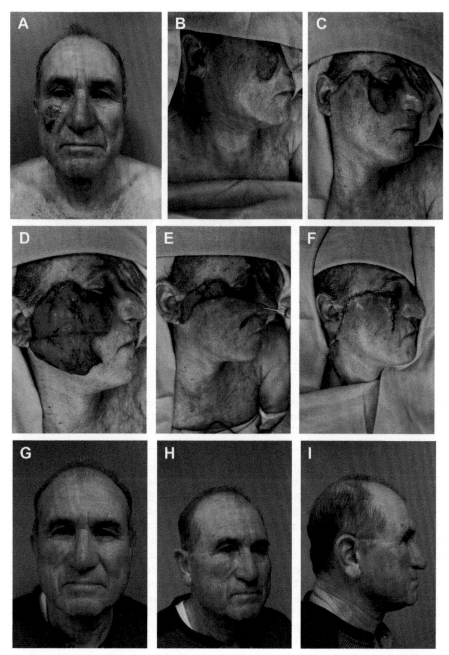

Fig. 6. Cervicofacial flap. (*A*) Melanoma of cheek status post margin-positive excision and full-thickness skin graft. (*B*) Full-thickness circular defect involving the right cheek. (*C*) Inferiorly based cervicofacial flap incised along the cheek-lid junction toward the outer canthus, the temple and temporal hairline, and the preauricular skin inferiorly to the tragus. (*D*) Flap elevated in subcutaneous plane and reflected. (*E*, *F*) Flap is rotated and inset into the defect over a drain. Distal flap tip ischemia related to local vasoconstrictive agent injection resolved spontaneously. (*G–I*) Postoperative results at 6 months.

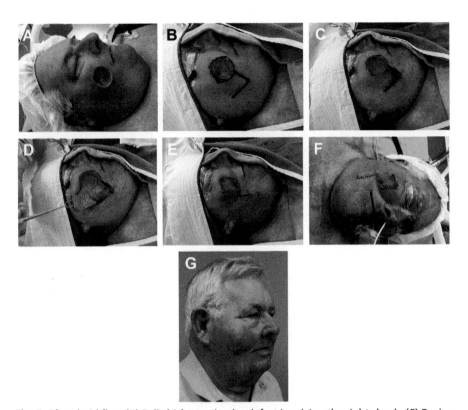

Fig. 7. Rhomboid flap. (*A*) Full-thickness circular defect involving the right cheek. (*B*) Design of inferiorly based rhomboid flap. (*C, D*) Flap incised, elevated in a subcutaneous plane, and reflected. (*E, F*) Flap inset and closure. (*G*) Postoperative results at 4 weeks.

The bilobed flap is yet another transposition flap that is particularly useful in nasal reconstruction, because lax tissues from the upper two-thirds of the nose are used to reconstruct defects in the less mobile lower-third (**Fig. 8**). The bilobed flap is a double transposition flap consisting of two lobes based on the same pedicle designed along a circular arc. First, the arc of rotation for the entire flap is marked from the distal edge of the wound. Next, a pivot point is placed about one radius away from the opposing wound edge and a Burow triangle is designed from this point to excise the intervening tissue between the pivot point and the defect. The first lobe is then designed identical in size to the defect at a 45° angle from the pivot point along the circular arc. The second lobe, which is designed narrower, longer, and with a triangular tip, is then placed at a 90° angle from the pivot point.[34,35] After flap design is completed, the Burow triangle is excised and the flap is raised in a subcutaneous or submuscular plane and rotated 45° into the defect.[35] The defect is closed with the first lobe, the primary donor site is closed with the second lobe, and the secondary donor site is closed primarily.

Axial flaps

An exhaustive description of all flaps with axial pattern, or named, blood supply exceeds the scope of this article. A sampling of common and pertinent pedicled axial flaps for oncologic cutaneous reconstruction follows.

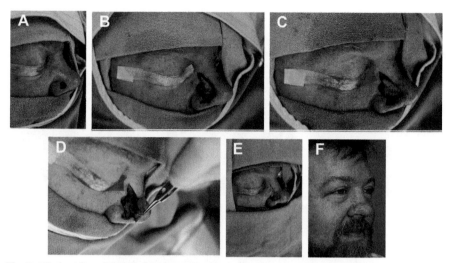

Fig. 8. Bilobed flap. (*A*) Full-thickness circular defect involving the right nasal ala. (*B*) Design of bilobed flap with anteriorly based pivot point. (*C–E*) Flap incised, elevated in a subcutaneous plane, and transposed into the defect without effacement of alar crease. (*F*) Postoperative results at 6 weeks.

Forehead flap The paramedian forehead flap, as described by Menick,[36] is a reliable flap to reconstruct nasal tip, lobule, and ala defects, or for even larger subtotal or total nasal reconstructions (**Fig. 9**). The flap provides large amounts of tissue with favorable color and texture match. Its blood supply is the supratrochlear pedicle, which originates deep to the medial brow about 1.7 to 2.2 cm from the midline and travels superiorly at varying tissue depths.[37] Preoperative assessment of vertical forehead dimensions, hairline position, defect size, and exposed or missing nasal structures is paramount. The length of available forehead tissue should be measured from the pivot point at the medial brow through the arc of rotation. The templated defect may be traced at the superior forehead along the path of the Doppler-confirmed vascular pedicle. The flap is elevated in the subcutaneous, subgaleal, and subperiosteal planes sequentially from distal to proximal. After inset, the flap remains pedicled for 3 to 4 weeks. Donor defects are partially left to heal by secondary intention with good cosmesis.[5] Patients should be counseled about postoperative wound care, multiple surgical stages, and the temporarily unappealing appearance before pedicle division. Secondary revisions for flap thinning are not uncommon.

Nasolabial flap The nasolabial flap is another reliable option for the reconstruction of smaller nasal defects of the sidewall and ala with intact lining (**Fig. 10**). Suitable candidates include patients with sufficient cheek laxity and well-defined nasolabial folds.[38] The superiorly based nasolabial flap is based on retrograde flow through the angular artery. In designing the flap, the medial edge overlies the nasolabial fold and the lateral extent is dictated by the width of the defect. The flap length is determined by assessing the arc of rotation from the intended pivot point. The flap may also be based inferiorly off of the facial artery.

Propeller flaps Emerging over the last decade, the propeller flap was originally conceived for reconstruction of defects in the distal one-third of the leg, a region with scant amount of lax tissues usually requiring free flap reconstruction.[39] It is a

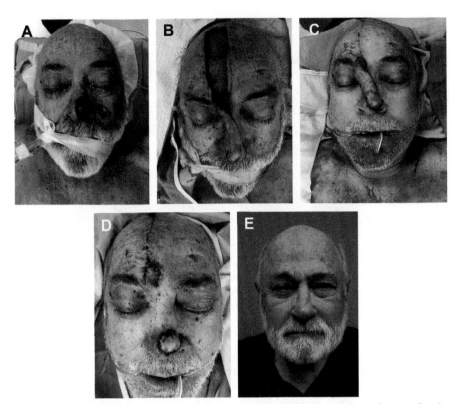

Fig. 9. Forehead flap. (*A*) Circular defect involving multiple nasal aesthetic subunits, including the right nasal tip, soft triangle, and ala. (*B, C*) Contralateral forehead flap based on right supratrochlear vessels elevated at various depths and inset into defect with primary closure of donor site. (*D*) Second-stage procedure at 3 weeks for pedicle division. (*E*) Postoperative results at 6 months. Additional procedure for flap thinning was performed 3 months after second stage.

locoregional island fasciocutaneous flap based on a single off-center perforating branch that branches off of a main named pedicle. The off-center perforator, which serves as the pivot point, splits up the flap tissues into two blades of unequal length. The longer arm is placed more proximally, so that when the flap is fully elevated and rotated 180°, the longer arm covers the defect. The shorter arm covers the donor site, which sometimes requires adjunctive skin grafting (**Fig. 11**).

Although propeller flaps are appealing alternatives to free flaps, they are technically difficult surgeries with high rates of partial flap loss (11.3%) and venous congestion (8.1%), and represent an advanced form of reconstruction.[40] As technical refinements have been made with increased experience, propeller flaps have become more popular and the indications have expanded to include upper extremity and truncal reconstruction.

Pedicled and free muscle, myocutaneous, and fasciocutaneous flaps

Larger and more complex three-dimensional defects after wide local excision require early involvement of a reconstructive surgeon. These complicated cases often require either larger pedicled flaps from regional tissues or free flaps from distant sites. Although uncommon in the context of reconstruction for melanoma-related defects,

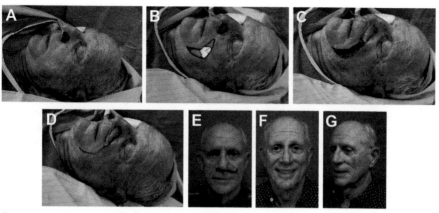

Fig. 10. Nasolabial flap. (*A*) Full-thickness defect extending from the left nasal ala to the medial cheek. (*B*) Nasolabial flap designed extending laterally from the nasolabial fold using a suture foil template of the defect. (*C, D*) Flap incised and inset into defect with primary closure of donor site. (*E*) Two weeks postoperative appearance with skin bridge intact. (*F, G*) The skin bridge was divided at 2 weeks and flap inset completed. Additional flap thinning procedures were undertaken. Postoperative results at 6 months after index procedure are depicted.

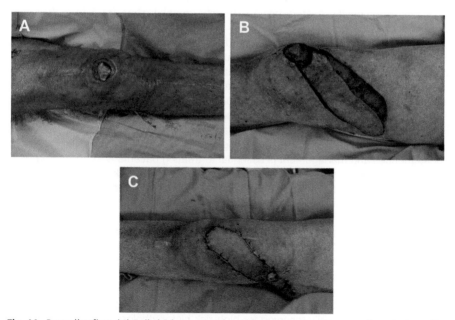

Fig. 11. Propeller flap. (*A*) Full-thickness circular defect extending down to denuded patella. (*B*) Superomedially based thigh propeller flap incised and elevated in subcutaneous plane down to fascia. Perforator dissected for adequate length to facilitate rotation. (*C*) Flap inset and donor site closure following 180° rotation of the flap. A small full-thickness skin graft was used for adjunctive donor site closure.

the use of these advanced techniques may become necessary in scenarios that involve recurrent disease, reoperation where local options have been exhausted, radiated fields, and loss of or exposure of critical anatomy. Reconstructive considerations are not limited to primary melanoma resection sites, but also at locations of regional lymphadenectomy. Patient comorbidities and functional status should be taken into account.

There are various types of pedicled and free flaps, including muscle, fascial, fasciocutaneous, bony, and composite flaps. Many of these flaps can be transferred as pedicled or free flaps, depending on the reconstructive needs and the location of the defect. Some common examples include the pectoralis major, latissimus dorsi, rectus abdominis, radial forearm, and anterolateral thigh flaps.

POSTOPERATIVE CARE

Meticulous postoperative care and follow-up is an invaluable adjunct to thorough preoperative planning and successful intraoperative execution. Skin graft postoperative care aims to ensure appropriate graft adherence to the recipient bed. Although various postoperative care regimens are described in the literature, most aim to facilitate compression of the graft against the recipient bed to prevent seroma or hematoma. A bolster dressing may be used to secure the graft. Negative pressure wound therapy is useful in exudative, irregular, or mobile and functional recipient sites to promote graft adherence.[41] As an adjunct to graft healing, wound vac therapy has been shown to provide a secure dressing that decreases bacterial counts, improves graft survival, and minimizes the need for repeat grafting.[42]

Postoperative activity is an important consideration, especially in extremity reconstruction. Traditionally, postoperative extremity immobilization for 5 to 7 days has been standard. However, immobilization is associated with increased morbidity, such as decreased range of motion, deconditioning, increased rates of thromboembolism, and longer hospitalizations. Recent studies have shown similar rates of skin graft take with early or even immediate ambulation.[43] The postoperative activity regimen should be tailored to the specific reconstruction, because certain body parts, such as the sole of the foot, benefit from immobilization.[44]

A high incidence of postoperative lymphedema has been reported following sentinel lymph node biopsy and completion or therapeutic lymph node dissection after melanoma wide local excision.[45] As such, having a general understanding of lymphedema consequences and management is essential to treating patients with melanoma. The main risks associated with lymphedema are increased rates of skin and soft tissue infections; lymphangitis; and rarely, lymphangiosarcoma. Furthermore, it can have negative psychological and social impacts on patients.[46] Preventive measures, including weight management and supervised exercise programs, have been shown to decrease the risk of lymphedema development.[47] For those who develop lymphedema, prompt referral for decongestive therapy is the gold standard.[48] In refractory cases, surgical intervention, such as volume-reduction procedures, lymphovenous bypass, and node transfers, may be considered.

The indications for adjuvant therapies in melanoma are extensive and evolving as new modalities are developed. Although the guidelines for radiation therapy are not well-defined, it is generally reserved for high-risk histopathologic features. Radiation consequences on reconstructions are well-described and include delayed wound healing issues, scar contractures, volume loss, and decreased skin integrity and tissue vascularity.[49] Furthermore, when adjuvant radiation is directed at the nodal basins, there is an even higher risk of lymphedema.[50]

SUMMARY

Wide local excision of melanoma remains the standard of care. In addressing the resultant complex defects, there is a wide range of tools within the reconstructive armamentarium. Each reconstruction should aim to restore form and function while minimizing donor site morbidity and preserving oncologic treatment efficacy. By working alongside surgical and medical oncologists, the reconstructive surgeon serves as an integral member of the melanoma multidisciplinary oncologic team.

DISCLOSURE

The authors have nothing to disclose.

REFERENCES

1. Moncrieff M. Excision margins for melanomas: how wide is enough? Lancet Oncol 2016;17(2):127–8.
2. NCCN Clinical Practice Guidelines in Oncology. Cutaneous Melanoma Web site. 2019. Available at: https://www.nccn.org/professionals/physician_gls/pdf/cutaneous_melanoma.pdf. Accessed July 15, 2019.
3. Hwang K, Lee JP, Yoo SY, et al. Relationships of comorbidities and old age with postoperative complications of head and neck free flaps: a review. J Plast Reconstr Aesthet Surg 2016;69(12):1627–35.
4. Janis JE, Kwon RK, Lalonde DH. A practical guide to wound healing. Plast Reconstr Surg 2010;125(6):230e–44e.
5. Meaike JD, Dickey RM, Killion E, et al. Facial skin cancer reconstruction. Semin Plast Surg 2016;30(3):108–21.
6. Bogle M, Kelly P, Shenaq J, et al. The role of soft tissue reconstruction after melanoma resection in the head and neck. Head Neck 2001;23(1):8–15.
7. Rinker B. The evils of nicotine: an evidence-based guide to smoking and plastic surgery. Ann Plast Surg 2013;70(5):599–605.
8. Barlow RJ, White CR, Swanson NA. Mohs' micrographic surgery using frozen sections alone may be unsuitable for detecting single atypical melanocytes at the margins of melanoma in situ. Br J Dermatol 2002;146(2):290–4.
9. Smith-Zagone MJ, Schwartz MR. Frozen section of skin specimens. Arch Pathol Lab Med 2005;129(12):1536–43.
10. Parrett BM, Kashani-Sabet M, Leong SP, et al. The safety of and indications for immediate reconstruction of head and neck melanoma defects: our early experience. Ann Plast Surg 2014;72(Suppl 1):S35–7.
11. Sullivan SR, Scott JR, Cole JK, et al. Head and neck malignant melanoma: margin status and immediate reconstruction. Ann Plast Surg 2009;62(2):144–8.
12. Thomas JR, Frost TW. Immediate versus delayed repair of skin defects following resection of carcinoma. Otolaryngol Clin North Am 1993;26(2):203–13.
13. Quimby AE, Khalil D, Johnson-Obaseki S. Immediate versus delayed reconstruction of head and neck cutaneous melanoma. Laryngoscope 2018;128(11):2566–72.
14. Moncrieff MD, Thompson JF, Quinn MJ, et al. Reconstruction after wide excision of primary cutaneous melanomas: part I-the head and neck. Lancet Oncol 2009;10(7):700–8.
15. Robinson JK. Segmental reconstruction of the face. Dermatol Surg 2004;30(1):67–74.

16. Eskiizmir G, Baker S, Cingi C. Nonmelanoma skin cancer of the head and neck: reconstruction. Facial Plast Surg Clin North Am 2012;20(4):493–513.

17. Wei FC, Mardini S. Flaps and reconstructive surgery. 1st edition. Philadelphia: Elsevier; 2009.

18. Moncrieff MD, Thompson JF, Quinn MJ, et al. Reconstruction after wide excision of primary cutaneous melanomas: part II–the extremities. Lancet Oncol 2009; 10(8):810–5.

19. Mathes SJ, Nahai F. Clinical applications for muscle and musculocutaneous flaps. St. Louis, MO: Mosby, Incorporated; 1982.

20. Janis JE, Kwon RK, Attinger CE. The new reconstructive ladder: modifications to the traditional model. Plast Reconstr Surg 2011;127(Suppl 1):205s–12s.

21. Fazio MJ, Zitelli JA. Principles of reconstruction following excision of nonmelanoma skin cancer. Clin Dermatol 1995;13(6):601–16.

22. Adams DC, Ramsey ML. Grafts in dermatologic surgery: review and update on full- and split-thickness skin grafts, free cartilage grafts, and composite grafts. Dermatol Surg 2005;31(8 Pt 2):1055–67.

23. McGregor IA, Morgan G. Axial and random pattern flaps. Br J Plast Surg 1973; 26(3):202–13.

24. Milton SH. Pedicled skin-flaps: the fallacy of the length: width ratio. Br J Surg 1970;57(7):502–8.

25. Krishnan R, Garman M, Nunez-Gussman J, et al. Advancement flaps: a basic theme with many variations. Dermatol Surg 2005;31(8 Pt 2):986–94.

26. Behan FC. The keystone design perforator island flap in reconstructive surgery. ANZ J Surg 2003;73(3):112–20.

27. Moncrieff MD, Bowen F, Thompson JF, et al. Keystone flap reconstruction of primary melanoma excision defects of the leg-the end of the skin graft? Ann Surg Oncol 2008;15(10):2867–73.

28. Goldman GD. Rotation flaps. Dermatol Surg 2005;31(8 Pt 2):1006–13.

29. LoPiccolo MC. Rotation flaps-principles and locations. Dermatol Surg 2015; 41(Suppl 10):S247–54.

30. Juri J, Juri C. Advancement and rotation of a large cervicofacial flap for cheek repairs. Plast Reconstr Surg 1979;64(5):692–6.

31. Crow ML, Crow FJ. Resurfacing large cheek defects with rotation flaps from the neck. Plast Reconstr Surg 1976;58(2):196–200.

32. Rohrer TE, Bhatia A. Transposition flaps in cutaneous surgery. Dermatol Surg 2005;31(8 Pt 2):1014–23.

33. Limberg AA. Modern trends in plastic surgery. Design of local flaps. Mod Trends Plast Surg 1966;2:38–61.

34. Zitelli JA. The bilobed flap for nasal reconstruction. Arch Dermatol 1989;125(7): 957–9.

35. Cook JL. A review of the bilobed flap's design with particular emphasis on the minimization of alar displacement. Dermatol Surg 2000;26(4):354–62.

36. Menick FJ. Aesthetic refinements in use of forehead for nasal reconstruction: the paramedian forehead flap. Clin Plast Surg 1990;17(4):607–22.

37. Shumrick KA, Smith TL. The anatomic basis for the design of forehead flaps in nasal reconstruction. Arch Otolaryngol Head Neck Surg 1992;118(4):373–9.

38. Bi H, Xing X, Li J. Nasolabial-alar crease: a natural line to facilitate transposition of the nasolabial flap for lower nasal reconstruction. Ann Plast Surg 2014;73(5): 520–4.

39. Teo TC. The propeller flap concept. Clin Plast Surg 2010;37(4):615–26, vi.

40. Gir P, Cheng A, Oni G, et al. Pedicled-perforator (propeller) flaps in lower extremity defects: a systematic review. J Reconstr Microsurg 2012;28(9):595–601.

41. Molnar JA, DeFranzo AJ, Marks MW. Single-stage approach to skin grafting the exposed skull. Plast Reconstr Surg 2000;105(1):174–7.

42. Scherer LA, Shiver S, Chang M, et al. The vacuum assisted closure device: a method of securing skin grafts and improving graft survival. Arch Surg 2002; 137(8):930–3 [discussion: 933–4].

43. Gawaziuk JP, Peters B, Logsetty S. Early ambulation after-grafting of lower extremity burns. Burns 2018;44(1):183–7.

44. Liu HH, Chang CK, Huang CH, et al. Use of split-thickness plantar skin grafts in the management of leg and foot skin defects. Int Wound J 2018;15(5):783–8.

45. Moody JA, Botham SJ, Dahill KE, et al. Complications following completion lymphadenectomy versus therapeutic lymphadenectomy for melanoma: a systematic review of the literature. Eur J Surg Oncol 2017;43(9):1760–7.

46. Fu MR, Ridner SH, Hu SH, et al. Psychosocial impact of lymphedema: a systematic review of literature from 2004 to 2011. Psychooncology 2013;22(7):1466–84.

47. Ryan TJ. Lymphatics and adipose tissue. Clin Dermatol 1995;13(5):493–8.

48. Warren AG, Brorson H, Borud LJ, et al. Lymphedema: a comprehensive review. Ann Plast Surg 2007;59(4):464–72.

49. Yun JH, Diaz R, Orman AG. Breast reconstruction and radiation therapy. Cancer Control 2018;25(1). 1073274818795489.

50. Kan CE, Mansur DB. The role of radiation therapy in the management of cutaneous melanoma. Melanoma Manag 2016;3(1):61–72.

Age and Melanocytic Lesions

Adrienne B. Shannon, MD[a],*, Yun Song, MD[a], Xiaowei Xu, MD[b],
Giorgos C. Karakousis, MD[c]

KEYWORDS

- Pediatric melanoma • Adolescent melanoma • Spitz nevi
- Melanocytic lesions and age • Lymph node metastases

KEY POINTS

- Pediatric and adolescent melanocytic lesions and melanoma are rare and exhibit different presentations, histologic subtypes, and outcomes compared with adult lesions.
- Spitzoid melanocytic lesions represent a subtype of pediatric lesions that exhibit differences in presentation, histologic diagnosis, and surveillance and generally have improved outcomes compared with nonspitzoid melanoma.
- Increasing age is associated with a decreased incidence of lymph node metastases in patients with melanoma.
- Despite having lower rates of lymph node metastases, older patients frequently present with high-risk features of melanoma and often have a worse prognosis and worse outcomes compared with younger patients.

INTRODUCTION

Patient age is known to be an independent risk factor in melanoma for high-risk primary tumor features, lymph node (LN) metastases, and survival outcomes. From pediatric and adolescent disease to disease in the elderly, there are clear differences in disease features and treatment outcomes, although the etiology for these differences remain to be elucidated. Understanding how melanoma and other melanocytic lesions behave in these various age populations is important for clinicians in guiding the diagnosis, treating the patient, understanding the prognosis, and surveilling the disease.

[a] Department of Surgery, Hospital of the University of Pennsylvania, 3400 Spruce Street, 4 Maloney, Philadelphia, PA 19104, USA; [b] Department of Pathology and Laboratory Medicine, Hospital of the University of Pennsylvania, 3400 Spruce Street, 6 Founders, Philadelphia, PA 19104, USA; [c] Department of Surgery, Hospital of the University of Pennsylvania, 3400 Spruce Street, 4 Silverstein, Philadelphia, PA 19104, USA
* Corresponding author.
E-mail address: Adrienne.shannon@pennmedicine.upenn.edu
Twitter: @abruceshannon (A.B.S.)

Surg Oncol Clin N Am 29 (2020) 369–386
https://doi.org/10.1016/j.soc.2020.02.005
1055-3207/20/Published by Elsevier Inc.

Pediatric and Adolescent Melanoma

Pediatric or juvenile cutaneous melanoma is defined most commonly as melanoma that affects patients from birth through age 20 and usually is divided into pediatric or prepubertal cohorts (ages 0–10) and adolescent or pubertal cohorts (ages 10–20).[1,2] It is a childhood disease of relatively low incidence, accounting for 1% to 4% of melanomas nationwide, but is the most common solid tumor in patients aged 15 years to 29 years.[3] Similar to adult melanoma, juvenile cutaneous melanoma has witnessed, at least until recent years, an increase in incidence.[1,2,4–6] Between 1988 and 2007, Surveillance, Epidemiology and End Results (SEER) data noted an increase in incidence per year of 2% for pubertal patients and 1% in prepubertal patients.[2,4] Young adults (ages 20–24 years) and pubertal patients had a similar increase in incidence of cutaneous melanoma, approximately 3%/year, but prepubertal patients had an increase in incidence of only 1.4%/year.[1,2,5,6] Despite these findings, the Western Australian Melanoma Advisory Service (WAMAS)[7] noted a decline in the incidence of juvenile melanoma since 2000 and SEER data[8] from 2000 to 2010 support a decline in incidence in more recent years (**Table 1**). This decline in incidence may be due to increased sun exposure awareness and decreased tanning bed use worldwide.

Similar to their adult counterparts, juvenile patients with cutaneous melanoma are more likely to have had exposure to UV radiation as measured by time outdoors, family history of melanoma, Fitzpatrick skin type 3 or below, light hair color, immune suppression, history of prior malignancy, or history of multiple benign or atypical nevi based on 1973 to 2007 SEER data.[1,2,4,9] National Cancer Database (NCDB) data show that prepubertal patients diagnosed from 1985 to 2003 were more likely to be male,[10] but the Regional Quality Register of Cutaneous Malignant Melanoma (Sweden), US National Center for Health Statistics from 1968 to 2004, and WAMAS experience suggest that juvenile melanoma patients are more likely to be female, with the exception of ages 1 year to 4 years.[5,7,11] These gender differences historically are hypothesized to largely reflect cultural differences regarding sun and UV exposure.

Disease presentation for both prepubertal and pubertal melanoma differ compared with adult melanoma presentation. Although adult patients frequently present with lesions according to the traditional ABCDE criteria (asymmetry, irregular borders, varied colors, increased diameter, and evolution or change in the lesion) as reasons for concern for a melanocytic lesion, juvenile melanoma commonly present with atypical criteria.[12] In this population, most lesions are amelanotic, up to 50%, bleeding, raised, and uniform in color.[7,12–14] The most common presenting sign in this population is evolution "E" of the lesion; evolution was noted to exist in 50% of WAMAS-reported patients.[7] Juvenile melanoma patients have a higher incidence of thick melanoma at diagnosis, likely a result of their difference in presentation and challenges in diagnosis, and typically are later stage compared with young adult groups.[1,2,4,6,9,10,12,13,15–19] Nodular types are most common in juvenile patients in nationwide analysis, although institutional cohorts and international cohorts note superficial spreading as the most common subtype.[1,2,6,7,11,13,15,16,20] Juvenile patients exhibited a higher incidence of nonwhite race and head and neck primaries, particularly in patients ages 1 year to 4 years and male patients.[1,2,4] Lower extremity, particularly in female patients ages 1 year to 4 years of age, and truncal lesions were more common in single-institution studies.[7,10,11,13,15] Pubertal patients are more likely to be fair-skinned and have a history of many nevi.[7,10] Multiple small and large nevi, both congenital and noncongenital, increase the risk of developing melanoma in pediatric patients by 4-fold. This risk increases by12-fold if patients have more than 10 nevi.[13]

Table 1
Review of major population-based studies examining the incidence, characteristics, and outcomes of pediatric and adolescent melanoma spanning 1953 through 2011

Authors	Years of Study	Data Source	Patient Population	Incidence Trend	Higher Incidence Factors Overall	Age <10 y	Survival Differences	Predictors of Poor Survival
Averbrook et al,[22] 2013	1953–2008	Multi-institutional (12) study	365 total pediatric patients	No comment	Females Clark level IV	Males More mitoses	Overall 5YS 79.7% 100% patients ≤10 y of age 81% patients >10 y of age No significant difference in age groups	Lesions ≥1.01 mm Stage of disease Ulceration
Lewis,[5] 2008	1968–2004	US National Center for Health Statistics	643 deaths due to melanoma in children 0–19 y of age	Decreased mortality incidence (1.5%/y)	No comment	No comment	Mortality rate reported 2.25 deaths/y/10 million at-risk individuals	Adolescents (15–19 y of age) White Male
Strouse et al,[2] 2005	1973–2001	SEER	3898 total patients Patients <20 y of age (N = 1225) Patients 20–24 y (N = 2673)	Incidence increased (2.9%/year)	White Females Extremities	Nonwhite Nodular Head/face/neck Thicker lesions Prior cancer	Overall 5YS 96.1% local (88.9% <10 y; 91.5% 11–19 y) 77.2% regional 57.3% distant	Male Metastases Nodular Head/face/neck Prior cancer

(continued on next page)

Table 1
(continued)

Authors	Years of Study	Data Source	Patient Population	Incidence Trend	Higher Incidence Factors			Survival Differences	Predictors of Poor Survival
					Overall	Age <10 y			
Aldrink et al,[15] 2009	1973–2007	Institutional database (Duke University Medical Center)	150 total patients Prepubertal (0–11 y) (N = 16) Ages 12–16 y (N = 63) Ages 17–19 y (N = 71)	No comment	Female Superficial spreading	Thick lesions (≥2.01 mm)		OS 84%	Recurrence higher in black patients, patients 17–19 y, ocular melanoma, and lesions ≥4.01 mm
Lange et al,[10] 2007	1985–2003	NCDB	3158 total patients	No comment	No comment	Male Head and neck Metastases Thick lesions (≥1.50 mm)		Age-specific 5YS 77% 1–9 y of age No significant difference in age groups >10 y of age	Females 1–9 y Males ≥10 y Patients 1–19 y
Moore-Olufemi et al,[17] 2011	1992–2006	Institutional database (MD Anderson Cancer Center)	109 total patients Prepubertal patients (1–9 y) (N = 25) Pubertal patients (10–17 y) (N = 84)	No comment	White Female	Nonwhite Thick lesions (≥2.01 mm) Positive nodes Spitzoid lesion LVI		Overall 10YS 89% No significant difference in age groups	Positive nodes

Study	Years	Database	Number	Incidence		Poor prognosis	Survival	
Austin et al,[4] 2013	1998–2007	SEER	1447 total patients	Increased incidence (2.5%/y) Highest increase in adolescents (2%/y)	Female Adolescent (>10 y)	Nonwhite Extremity Head/neck Nodular Thick lesions (≥1.01 mm) Higher stage	No comment	No comment
Lorimer et al,[21] 2016	1998–2011	NCDB	3965 total patients Patients 1–10 y (N = 306) Patients 11–20 y (N = 3659)	No defined trend	White Males 1–10 y Females 11–20 y Head/neck if 1–10 y Trunk if 11–20 y	Thick lesion (T3/4) Positive nodes Head and neck	Age-specific 5YS 94.1% patients <10 y and node-positive 96% patients <10 y and node-negative	Adolescents (11–20 y) Males Black Positive nodes
Campbell et al,[8] 2015	2000–2010	SEER	1185 total patients	Decreased incidence (−11.58%/y)	White Superficial spreading Head/neck if 0–4 y Extremity if 5–9 y Trunk if 14–19 y	Ulceration Positive nodes Distant metastases	No comment	No comment
Lam et al,[18] 2018	2004–2008	SEER	1255 total patients Patients ≤12 y (N = 138) Patients 13–18 y (N = 456) Patients 19–21 y (N = 661)	No comment	White Trunk Superficial spreading	Higher stage (stage III/IV)	No comment	Age 19–21 y Black

Abbreviations: 5YS, 5-year survival; 10YS, 10-year survival; LVI, lymphovascular invasion.
Data from Refs.[2,4,5,8,10,15,17,18,21,22]

Similar to adults, Breslow thickness is associated with a significant increase in risk of metastasis in juvenile patients, and both SEER and single-institution studies demonstrate a direct relationship with survival outcomes.[2,12,14,18,20] Data from SEER demonstrate that prepubertal patients in particular are diagnosed at later stage with increased thickness lesions at presentation and subsequently demonstrate a worse survival.[18] These data show 5-year survival rates to be 96% for localized disease and 77% for regional disease, with evidence of increased survival at a rate of 4%/year over the previous 3 decades.[2,15] NCDB and single-institutional data suggest that despite increased thickness lesions at presentation, juvenile patients, in particular prepubertal patients, do not demonstrate a worse prognosis but rather have improved overall survival (OS) and recurrence-free survival when controlling for stage, thickness, and ulceration compared with adult patients, suggesting discordance between SEER and NCDB data.[10,11,15,20,21] Despite an improved prognosis in juvenile compared with adult patients, survival is overall worse in patients who are male, white, and prepubertal.[1,2,10,22,23] LN metastasis is more common in patients less than 10 years of age,[17,18,20,22,23] and data from SEER (2004–2008) indicate that patients less than 10 years of age have a higher rate of distant disease.[18] This may suggest an influence of hormones on melanoma tumor biology in the pediatric patient.

Age and Histopathology of Melanocytic Lesions and Melanoma

Pediatric melanomas are classified into 5 subtypes: conventional melanoma, spitzoid melanoma, melanoma arising in large and giant congenital melanocytic nevi (CMN), congenital melanoma, and leptomeningeal melanoma associated with neurocutaneous melanosis.[24] In addition to these 5 subtypes, there are melanocytic tumors of uncertain malignant potential (MelTUMPs).[24] MelTUMPs (**Fig. 1**), and their subtype, spitzoid melanocytic tumor of uncertain malignant potential (STUMPs), represent a diagnostic challenge for pathologists because there is little consensus on their diagnosis.[14,25,26] Conventional melanoma, accounting for 40% to 50% of pediatric melanomas, behaves similar to adult melanoma and traditionally is found in prepubertal, white patients with numerous nevi.[24] As in adult melanoma, BRAF mutations drive 85% of pediatric conventional melanomas.[24]

Although rare, 3 of the 5 pediatric subtypes are considered congenital. These 3, melanoma arising from CMN, congenital melanoma, and leptomeningeal melanoma, are associated with a poorer prognosis. In CMN, patients with either large (20–40 cm) and giant (>40 cm or >5% skin surface at birth) nevi have a 6% risk of malignant transformation. This phenotype is aggressive and rapidly progresses to fatality. CMN lesions often have small, round blue cells and many mitotic figures on histologic examination and often have an activation mutation in NRAS at codon 61.[24] Congenital melanoma is present at birth or presents early in life and is either primarily congenital, typically on the scalp, or metastatic (via transplacental passage), from maternal melanoma during fetal development. Leptomeningeal melanoma associated with neurocutaneous melanosis, an even rarer entity, involves lesions in the frontal and temporal lobes and is rapidly fatal.[24]

The remaining subtype, spitzoid melanocytic lesions, are a spectrum of lesions that encompass typical Spitz nevi, atypical Spitz nevi, STUMPs, and spitzoid melanoma, summarized in **Table 2**. Compared with nonspitzoid melanoma, spitzoid lesions exhibit improved OS and outcomes.[27] Within this spectrum, spitzoid melanoma is characterized by large (>10 mm), asymmetric, amelanotic (25%), or pigmented papule or nodule that has enlarged epithelioid or spindle cells and absent epidermis or epidermal effacement (**Fig. 2**).[24,28] They have a vertical deposition of melanocytes and wedge-shaped architecture, dense cellularity with irregular nests with poor or

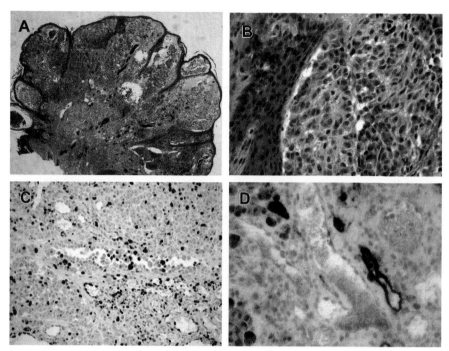

Fig. 1. Spitzoid MelTUMP identified from a 2-year-old boy. (A) Hematoxylin-eosin stain showing melanocytic lesion of uncertain malignant potential, original magnification ×40 (B) Hematoxylin-eosin stain showing melanocytic lesion of unknown malignant potential, original magnification ×400. (C) Ki67 staining shows increased proliferation in the tumor. (D) S-100 and D2-40 double staining shows melanoma cells in the lymphatic vessels.

absent maturation, and deep mitotic figures and high mitotic rate (>6 mitoses/mm).[24,29] They can be identified more often in prepubertal children than in pubertal children, but, when identified in pubertal children, often have an unpredictable clinical course.[24,29] Prepubertal children with spitzoid melanoma often lack risk factors and present with de novo, ulcerated lesions on the extremities or head.[28] Spitzoid melanomas are associated with single-nucleotide variations affecting the telomerase reverse transcriptase (TERT) promoter or activating BRAF protooncogene or chromosomal rearrangements, especially in pubertal patients.[14,28] They are associated with a high rate of LN metastasis (50%) but rarely are associated with distant disease unless a homozygous 9p21 deletion is present.[24,26,30] When associated with nodal metastasis, OS is superior to nonspitzoid melanoma, particularly in younger patients.[14,24]

Spitz nevi, initially described as benign juvenile melanoma in 1948, are melanocytic neoplasms containing epithelioid and spindle cells in patients under the age of 35 years of age but more commonly are associated with pediatric patients.[31] Of these lesions, at least half of all incidence occur in patients less than 10 years of age.[31] Spitz nevi are classically broken up into 2 classifications, typical and atypical. These lesions, compared with melanoma, are more associated with kinase fusion mutations, activating mutations in HRAS, loss of BAP1, chromosomal copy changes, and TERT promoter mutation; BRAF mutations are less likely to occur in association with these lesions.[24,32] In distinguishing between typical and atypical nevi, normal findings based on comparative genomic hybridization are reassuring, but additional testing based on

Table 2
Comparative summary of spitzoid lesions, including typical Spitz nevi, atypical Spitz nevi, and Spitz melanoma by disease presentation, histologic features, proliferative activity, and additional features based on systematic review of current pathologic literature

	Typical Spitz Nevus	Atypical Spitz Nevus	Spitz Melanoma
Presentation			
Age	Often <20 y, pubertal and prepubertal	Most often pubertal patients	Rare in prepubertal patients
Site	Often extremity and head/neck	Any	Any
Diameter	Small, <6 mm	>6 mm	Large, >10 mm
Border	Symmetric, wedge-shaped	Asymmetric	Asymmetric
Circumscription	Well circumscribed	Poorly circumscribed	Poorly circumscribed
Pigment	Even color superficially	Varied	Varied
Histology			
Cell type	Uniform epithelioid and spindle cells	Atypical epithelioid and spindle cells	Dense and enlarged epithelioid and spindle cells, increased atypia and pleomorphism
Cytoplasm	Clear, eosinophilic	Dusty, granular	Granular
Nuclei and nuclei	Uniform with delicate pattern	Heterogeneous and hyperchromasia, large	Hyperchromasia, large
Nuclear/cytoplasmic ratio	Low	Bordering on high	High
Epidermal hyperplasia	Present, uniform	Epidermal effacement, pagetoid spreading	Absent
Maturation/subcutaneous ext.	Present, ordered bordering of subcutaneous layer	Absent, subcutaneous extension evenly present	Poor or absent maturation, irregular vertical deposits of melanocytes
Ulceration	Absent	Present	Present
Kamino bodies	Present	Absent	Absent
Proliferative activity			
Mitotic activity	Absent or <2 mit/mm2	2–6 mm^2	>6 mit/mm^2
Proliferative index	<2%	2%–10%	>10%

(continued on next page)

Table 2
(continued)

	Typical Spitz Nevus	Atypical Spitz Nevus	Spitz Melanoma
Mutations	Uncommon; kinase fusion mutations, activating HRAS mutation, loss of BAP1, TERT mutations, chromosomal copy creation	Chromosomal deletions, including homozygous 9p21 deletion; chromosomal copies, including 11q13 gain	TERT mutations; BRAF activation; chromosome deletions, including homozygous 9p21 deletion
Other	Intact junctional clefts	Lack junctional clefts	

Data from Refs.[14,24–37]

fluorescence in situ hybridization is limited in its diagnostic discrimination in pediatric patients compared with adults.[14,33,34]

Typical Spitz nevi are solitary, small (<6 mm), and symmetric with even superficial pigment distribution and have uniform epidermal hyperplasia, maturation deep in the epidermis, and, entering the dermis, intact junctional clefts, uniform nucleoli with a clear eosinophilic cytoplasm, and absent or low mitotic activity (**Fig. 3**).[14,35] These lesions most often are well-circumscribed, pigmented or amelanotic papules or nodules.[31,32] Typical Spitz nevi exhibit a rapid growth phase followed by a static phase and can occur spontaneously or in conjunction with a preexisting melanocytic

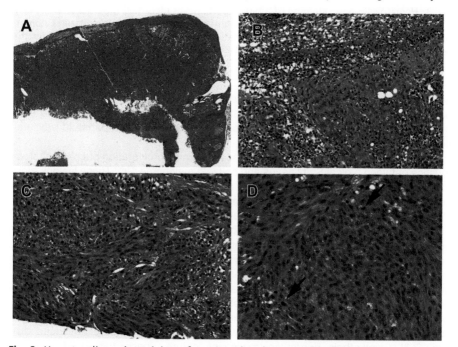

Fig. 2. Hematoxylin-eosin staining of a spitzoid melanoma identified from a 16-year-old boy. (A) Low-power view of lesion, original magnification ×40. (B) Ulcerated epidermis, original magnification ×400. (C) Lack of maturation from superficial to deep in the lesion, original magnification ×400. (D) Frequent mitoses (arrows), original magnification ×400..

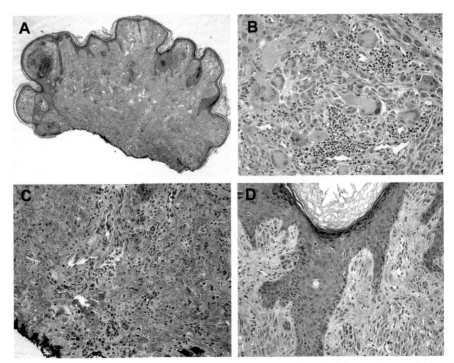

Fig. 3. Hematoxylin-eosin staining of a typical Spitz nevus identified from a 5-year-old boy. (A) Symmetric melanocytic lesion, original magnification ×40. (B) Typical spitzoid cytomorphology, original magnification ×400. (C) Maturation shown as the nevus cells enter the reticular dermis, original magnification ×400. (D) Focal pagetoid proliferation in the epidermis is allowed, original magnification ×400. .

nevus.[31] Often, their benign nature is indicated most strongly by the presence of large, pale eosinophilic Kamino bodies.[14,32] Histologically, typical Spitz nevi show a starburst or globular pattern with reticular depigmentation and limited pagetoid proliferation in the epidermis.[32]

In contrast, atypical Spitz nevi are lesions that exhibit proliferation but have characteristics between typical Spitz nevus and spitzoid melanoma.[31,35] These lesions most often are classified as malignant, but they are associated with minimal lethal potential compared with spitzoid and nonspitzoid melanoma.[31,35,36] They typically exhibit deep mitoses and focal necrosis, a pagetoid spread in the upper epidermis, heterogeneity of organization, and absence of Kamino bodies.[35,37] They are more similar to melanoma in that they exhibit variable pigment and asymmetry. Atypical Spitz nevi rarely have a glomerular structure and have an ulcerated epidermis, dense cellularity that lacks junctional clefts, hyperchromatism, large and eosinophilic nuclei, high nucleoli-to-cytoplasm ratio, and dusty/granular cytoplasm.[32,35] Pediatric patients, in particular, are likely to have increased mitotic rate and a greater likelihood of ulceration with these lesions.[25] These lesions often are associated with homozygous 9p21 deletions and 11q13 gains, which portend worse prognosis and more advanced disease.[26,30] Given their borderline malignant nature, these tumors do require complete excision and careful biannual to annual follow-up, although there does not appear to be a clear role for sentinel LN biopsy (SLNB), as expected in the management of melanoma.[14,26,32,36]

Age and Lymph Node Metastasis

Although patient age is not highlighted in the National Comprehensive Cancer Network (NCCN)[38] or the American Society of Clinical Oncology/Society of Surgical Oncology[39] clinical practice guidelines for SLNB, the inverse trend between age and the incidence of LN metastasis has been well documented. Increasing age has been associated with decreased rates of microscopic nodal disease in multiple retrospective institutional and population-based studies.[40–54] In the Sunbelt Melanoma Trial, which included 3076 patients with clinically node-negative melanoma greater than or equal to 1.0 mm in Breslow thickness who underwent SLNB, age under 30 years was associated with a significantly higher rate of sentinel LN (SLN) positivity.[40,41] Compared with patients older than 30 years, those 30 years or younger experienced an increased odds of SLN metastasis of 1.770 (95% CI, 1.260–2.486; P = .001).[41] The effect on SLN positivity appeared to start after age 40 and was more pronounced with increasing age.[40] Using the American Joint Committee on Cancer (AJCC) staging database of 7756 patients, Balch and colleagues[45] reported that patients younger than 20 years had an LN metastasis rate of 25.8%, whereas only 15.5% of those 80 years or older had metastatic LNs (P<.001).

Studies stratifying risk of nodal positivity using national databases have generally found age to be significant factor.[47,48,51,52,54] Using the NCDB, Conic and colleagues[48] evaluated the association between age and microscopic nodal disease in patients with clinically node-negative, thin melanoma who underwent regional LN surgery. Compared with those younger than 30 years, patients 70 years or older were significantly less likely to have LN metastases (odds ratio 0.56; 95% CI, 0.38–0.84). In a similar population of patients with thin melanoma from the NCDB, Sinnamon and colleagues[47] were able to stratify risk of nodal disease based on the presence of mitoses, primary tumor depth, and patient age. The highest-risk group had a rate of LN positivity of 6.5% (95% CI, 5.5%–7.6%) and were characterized by the presence of mitoses, tumor greater than or equal to 0.76 mm in thickness, and age younger than 65 years. Similarly, other studies using the NCDB have found that age, along with the presence of lymphovascular invasion, were significant determinants of SLN positivity in patients with intermediate thickness melanoma.[51,52] Specifically, in 1 study using NCDB data of patients with intermediate-thickness melanoma without primary tumor ulceration, every decade over 50 years corresponded to an allowance of an additional 0.5 mm in tumor depth over 1.0 mm while still maintaining a rate of SLN positivity under 5%, a threshold risk generally accepted to justify the performance of SLNB.[38,39,52] Although increasing age also has been associated with decreasing odds of SLN metastasis even in patients with thick melanoma, the overall rates of nodal disease in this patient population are very high,[53–57] with virtually all subgroups of patients, regardless of age and other clinical and tumor factors, exceeding 5% risk of nodal positivity.[54]

Distant Metastasis and Survival

Despite the inverse relationship between age and LN metastasis, older patients with melanoma experience worse survival outcomes. Although older patients typically have melanomas with higher-risk features, such as thicker tumors at the time of presentation, increased incidence of ulceration, and higher mean mitotic rates,[40,46,58–61] these tumor characteristics do not fully explain the observation of increased distant metastases and decreased survival in these patients.

Multiple studies have found age to be independently associated with distant disease-free survival (DFS), melanoma-specific survival (MSS), and/or OS, despite adjusting for primary tumor characteristics.[43,44,53,55–59] Among patients included in the AJCC staging database, MSS rates decreased gradually by increasing age, even when stratified by AJCC stage.[59] Egger and colleagues[44] reported that, in the subgroup of patients included in the Sunbelt Melanoma Trial with superficial spreading melanoma, ages 60 years or older were associated with worse OS (risk ratio 1.77; 95% CI, 1.39–2.25; $P<.0001$) compared with younger patients, even after adjusting for other important prognostic factors. Unlike other studies[53,55]; however, older age was not associated with a decrease in DFS (risk ratio 1.13; 95% CI, 0.84–1.49; $P = .4207$) in this study. The association between age and survival may differ by the status of the regional LN basin. In a study of SLNB in patients with thick melanoma, age was associated with OS in patients who were SLN-negative (hazard ratio [HR] 1.04; 95% CI, 1.01–1.06; $P = .0074$) but not in those with nodal metastases.

Several explanations have been offered to rationalize the difference in clinical outcomes observed by age in patients with melanoma. One such explanation from Ribero and colleagues[62] suggested that melanomas in an older patient may exhibit a different biologic behavior, particularly in those patients with a history of nevi. The presence of multiple nevi is a significant risk factor for developing melanoma. Nevi also are known to involute with senescence, and shortening of telomere length occurs with aging.[63] Despite being a risk factor for developing melanoma, a high nevus count was found associated with improved MSS (5-year rate 91.2% vs 86.5%; log-rank $P<.001$).[62]

In addition to differences in biologic behavior, melanomas in older patients may be influenced by remodeling of the host extracellular matrix that results in physical changes in the skin and impaired lymphatic vasculature that may be more favorable for the development of distant metastases. HAPLN1, a hyaluronic and proteoglycan link protein present in the extracellular matrix, is secreted in high levels by young dermal fibroblasts but lost in aged fibroblasts.[64] In studies by Kaur and colleagues[64] and Ecker and colleagues,[65] loss of HAPLN1 in fibroblasts in vitro resulted in an aligned extracellular matrix that was more favorable for melanoma metastasis and endothelial cells that had increased permeability. Using a mouse model for melanoma, Ecker and colleagues[65] further showed that aged mice developed fewer LN metastases but had a higher tumor burden in the lung, but reconstitution of HAPLN1 in these mice was able to reverse these observed clinical metastatic patterns. Finally, older patients who underwent SLNB for melanoma also demonstrated significantly lower radiotracer counts, a finding consistent with the notion of increased lymphovascular permeability with advanced age demonstrated in the in vitro and in vivo studies.[65] Together, these data support the hypothesis that changes within the extracellular matrix with age may produce an environment that decreases the containment of malignant cells within the lymphatic system and favors the development of distant metastases.

The Effect of Treatment and Age

Although older patients have an increased risk of melanoma-related death, they may be more likely to receive substandard surgical treatment[57,66] and offered adjuvant radiation and systemic therapies less frequently.[23] A population-based study of patients diagnosed with stages I to III melanoma found that age 65 years or older was independently associated with nonadherence to NCCN guidelines for surgical management, although the investigators could not account for comorbidities or other patient factors that may influence treatment decision making.[66]

Nevertheless, SLNB generally is considered a procedure with low morbidity,[67,68] and the procedure can be performed safely in older patients.[69] Moreover, LN status remains a significant prognostic factor in the elderly, in whom nodal positivity consistently has been associated with worse DFS and MSS.[69–71] In a 2-center retrospective study of patients age 70 years or older who underwent SLNB, the overall diagnostic accuracy was 98.0%.[69] Patients who had a positive SLN experienced worse 5-year DFS (39% vs 80%; log-rank $P<.001$) and MSS (46% vs 88.6%; log-rank $P<.001$). Adjusting for other prognostic factors, SLN status remained independently associated with MSS ($P<.001$), but increasing age beyond 70 years did not have an impact on MSS. Similarly, a single-institution study of 553 patients age 75 years or older reported that SLN positivity was associated with worse distant DFS (HR 2.61; 95% CI, 1.79–3.82; $P<.001$) and MSS (HR 3.75; 95% CI, 2.21–6.37; $P<.001$). Although age has an impact on the incidence of melanoma LN metastasis, elderly patients with a substantial risk of nodal disease and who are suitable candidates for surgery generally should be considered for SLNB according to guideline recommendations.

In the era of modern systemic therapies for melanoma, the question arises as to whether immune checkpoint inhibitors, which have become the standard of care in advanced melanoma, may be less efficacious in older patients as a result of immunosenescence or age-related alterations that lead to decreased immune function.[72,73] Yet, the data do not suggest that age is a strong factor influencing treatment efficacy.[74–77] In multicenter phase 3 trials that reported subgroup analyses by age, treatment with immune checkpoint inhibitors resulted in significant survival improvements in patients 65 years or older, just as in younger patients. Furthermore, the groups appear to experience similar rates of immune-related adverse events.[72]

These data suggest that treatment with immune checkpoint inhibitors can be safely considered in the elderly patient population. Elderly patients may demonstrate a greater survival advantage compared with their younger counterparts. Several investigations have shown that patients over the age of 60 respond more effectively to anti–PD-1 therapies, likely due to down-regulation of regulatory T cells.[78–80] Increasing age also has been shown to increase the response to anti–PD-1 therapy in patients with metastatic melanoma.[80]

SUMMARY

Age is an important factor to consider in the treatment of melanocytic lesions. Juvenile melanoma is a rare disease that has declined in incidence over the previous 2 decades but continues to represent a distinct disease entity. Pediatric patients with conventional cutaneous melanoma are more likely to present with thicker lesions and higher stage of disease. Despite this, their survival outcomes remain more favorable in comparison to adults. Aside from conventional disease, juvenile melanocytic lesions, including lesions of unknown malignant potential, Spitz nevi, and spitzoid melanoma, are distinct disease processes that have a spectrum of presentation and prognoses. Spitz lesions, although sometimes malignant, can be misdiagnosed as melanoma; careful pathologic evaluation of these lesions can help guide treatment and surveillance in juvenile patients.

Although juvenile melanocytic lesions have a relatively favorable prognosis, older age is associated with worse outcomes. Aging patients often present with more high-risk features that likely predispose them to a poorer prognosis, despite a lower incidence of LN metastases. This lower rate of LN metastasis and higher distant disease incidence may be attributable to changes in extracellular matrix proteins affecting lymphatic permeability and age-related differences in tumor biology. Given the relatively low morbidity of the SLNB procedure and its important prognostic role and implications for further therapy, this procedure should strongly be considered when indicated according to guidelines, even in older patients who are medically fit for surgery. Moreover, immune checkpoint inhibitors can be used safely in the elderly with significant response rates. When evaluating patients with melanocytic lesions, age should be an important consideration to help guide and inform the diagnosis, prognosis, and treatment of these patients.

DISCLOSURE

The authors have nothing to disclose.

REFERENCES

1. Sreeraman Kumar R, Messina JL, Reed D, et al. Pediatric melanoma and atypical melanocytic neoplasms. In: Kaufman H, Mehnert J, editors. Melanoma. Cancer treatment and research, vol. 167. Cham (Switzerland): Springer; 2016. p. 331–69.

2. Strouse JJ, Fears TR, Tucker MA, et al. Pediatric melanoma: risk factor and survival analysis of the surveillance, epidemiology, and end results database. J Clin Oncol 2005;23(21):4735–41.

3. Howlader N, Noone AM, Krapcho M, et al, editors. SEER cancer Statistics review, 1975-2016. Bethesda (MD): National Cancer Institute; 2019. based on November 2018 SEER data submission, posted to the SEER web site.

4. Austin MT, Xing Y, Hayes-Jordan AA, et al. Melanoma incidence rises for children and adolescents: an epidemiologic review of pediatric melanoma in the United States. J Pediatr Surg 2013;48(11):2207–13.

5. Lewis KG. Trends in pediatric melanoma mortality in the United States, 1968 through 2004. Dermatol Surg 2008;34(2):152–9.

6. Bagnoni G, Fidanzi C, Massimilliano A, et al. Melanoma in children, adolescents, and young adults: anatomoclinical features and prognostic study on 426 cases. Pediatr Surg Int 2019;35(1):159–65.

7. Xu JX, Koek S, Lee S, et al. Juvenile melanomas: Western Australian Melanoma Advisory Service experience. Australas J Dermatol 2017;58(4):299–303.

8. Campbell LB, Kreicher K, Gittleman HR, et al. Melanoma incidence in children and adolescents: decreasing trends in the United States. J Pediatr 2015;166:1505–13.

9. Livestro DP, Kaine EM, Michaelson JS, et al. Melanoma in the young: differences and similarities with adult melanoma: a case-matched controlled analysis. Cancer 2007;110(3):614–24.

10. Lange JR, Palis BE, Chang DC, et al. Melanoma in children and teenagers: an analysis of patients from the National Cancer Data Base. J Clin Oncol 2007;25(11):1363–8.

11. Plym A, Ullenhag GJ, Breivald M, et al. Clinical characteristics, management and survival in young adults diagnosed with malignant melanoma: A population-based cohort study. Acta Oncol 2014;53(5):688–96.

12. Cordoro KM, Gupta D, Frieden IJ, et al. Pediatric melanoma: results of a large cohort study and proposal for modified ABCD detection criteria for children. J Am Acad Dermatol 2013;68(6):913–25.

13. Ferrari A, Bono A, Baldi M, et al. Does melanoma behave differently in younger children than in adults? A retrospective study of 33 cases of childhood melanoma from a single institution. Pediatrics 2005;115(3):649–54.

14. Wood BA. Paediatric melanoma. Pathology 2016;48(2):155–65.

15. Aldrink JH, Selim MA, Diesen DL, et al. Pediatric melanoma: a single-institution experience of 150 patients. J Pediatr Surg 2009;44(8):1514–21.

16. Berk DR, LaBuz E, Dadras SS, et al. Melanoma and melanocytic tumors of uncertain malignant potential in children, adolescents, and young adults–the Stanford experience 1995-2008. Pediatr Dermatol 2010;27(3):244–54.
17. Moore-Olufemi S, Herzog C, Warneke C, et al. Outcomes in pediatric melanoma: comparing prepubertal to adolescent pediatric patients. Ann Surg 2011;253(6): 1211–5.
18. Lam PH, Obirieze AC, Ortega G, et al. An age-based analysis of pediatric melanoma: Staging, surgery, and mortality in the Surveillance, Epidemiology, and End Results database. Am Surg 2018;1(84):739–45.
19. Verzì AE, Bubley JA, Haugh AM, et al. A single-institution assessment of superficial spreading melanoma (SSM) in the pediatric population: Molecular and histopathologic features compared with adult SSM. J Am Acad Dermatol 2017;77(5): 886–92.
20. Pardela S, Fonseca E, Pita-Fernández S, et al. Prognostic factors for melanoma in children and adolescents: a clinicopathologic, single-center study of 137 patients. Cancer 2010;116:4334–44.
21. Lorimer PD, White RL, Walsh K, et al. Pediatric and adolescent melanoma: a national cancer data base update. Ann Surg Oncol 2016;23(12):4058–66.
22. Averbrook BJ, Lee SJ, Delman KA, et al. Pediatric melanoma: analysis of an international registry. Cancer 2013;119(22):4012–9.
23. Mu E, Lange JR, Strouse JJ. Comparison of the use and results of sentinel lymph node biopsy in children and young adults with melanoma. Cancer 2012;118(10): 2700–7.
24. Bahrami A, Barnhill RL. Pathology and genomics of pediatric melanoma: a critical reexamination and new insights. Pediatr Blood Cancer 2018;65(2). https://doi.org/10.1002/pbc.26792.
25. LaChance A, Shahriari M, Kerr PE, et al. Melanoma: Kids are not just little people. Clin Dermatol 2016;34(6):742–8.
26. McCormack L, Hawryluk EB. Pediatric melanoma update. G Ital Dermatol Venereol 2018;153(5):707–15.
27. Bailey KM, Durham AB, Zhao L, et al. Pediatric melanoma and aggressive Spitz tumors: a retrospective diagnostic, exposure and outcome analysis. Transl Pediatr 2018;7(3):203–10.
28. Carrera C, Scope A, Dusza SW, et al. Clinical and dermoscopic characterization of pediatric and adolescent melanomas: multicenter study of 52 cases. J Am Acad Dermatol 2018;78(2):278–88.
29. Bartenstein DW, Kelleher CM, Friedmann AM, et al. Contrasting features of childhood and adolescent melanomas. Pediatr Dermatol 2018;35(3):354–60.
30. Gerami P, Cooper C, Bajaj S, et al. Outcomes of atypical spitz tumors with chromosomal copy number aberrations and conventional melanomas in children. Am J Surg Pathol 2013;37(9):1387–94.
31. Abboud J, Stein M, Ramien M, et al. The diagnosis and management of Spitz nevus in the pediatric population: a systematic review and meta-analysis protocol. Syst Rev 2017;6(1):81.
32. Bartenstein DW, Fisher JM, Stamoulis C, et al. Clinical features and outcomes of spitzoid proliferations in children and adolescents. Br J Dermatol 2019;181(2): 366–72.
33. Dika E, Fanti PA, Fiorentino M, et al. Spitzoid tumors in children and adults: a comparative clinical, pathological, and cytogenetic analysis. Melanoma Res 2015;25(4):295–301.
34. Tracy ET, Aldrink JH. Pediatric melanoma. Semin Pediatr Surg 2016;25(5):290–8.

35. Paradela S, Fonseca E, Prieto VG. Melanoma in children. Arch Pathol Lab Med 2011;135(3):307–16.
36. Massi D, Tomasini C, Senetta R, et al. Atypical Spitz tumors in patients younger than 18 years. J Am Acad Dermatol 2015;71(1):37–46.
37. Tom WL, Hsu JW, Eichenfield LF, et al. Pediatric "STUMP" lesions: evaluation and management of difficult atypical Spitzoid lesions in children. J Am Acad Dermatol 2011;64(3):559–72.
38. Coit DG, Thompson JF, Albertini MR, et al. Cutaneous melanoma, version 2.2019, NCCN clinical practice guidelines in oncology. J Natl Compr Canc Netw 2019;17(4):367–402. Available at: https://www.nccn.org/professionals/physician_gls/default.aspx. Accessed March 15, 2019.
39. Wong SL, Faries MB, Kennedy EB, et al. Sentinel lymph node biopsy and management of regional lymph nodes in melanoma: American Society of Clinical Oncology and Society of Surgical Oncology clinical practice guideline update. Ann Surg Oncol 2018;25(2):356–77.
40. Chao C, Martin RCG II, Ross MI, et al. Correlation between prognostic factors and increasing age in melanoma. Ann Surg Oncol 2004;11(3):259–64.
41. Chagpar RB, Ross MI, Reintgen DS, et al. Factors associated with improved survival among young adult melanoma patients despite a greater incidence of sentinel lymph node metastasis. J Surg Res 2007;143(1):164–8.
42. Sassen S, Shaw HM, Colman MH, et al. The complex relationships between sentinel node positivity, patient age, and primary tumor desmoplasia: analysis of 2303 melanoma patients treated at a single center. Ann Surg Oncol 2008; 15(2):630–7.
43. Kretschmer L, Starz H, Thoms K-M, et al. Age as a key factor influencing metastasizing patterns and disease-specific survival after sentinel lymph node biopsy for cutaneous melanoma. Int J Cancer 2011;129(6):1435–42.
44. Egger ME, Stepp LO, Callender GG, et al. Outcomes and prognostic factors in superficial spreading melanoma. Am J Surg 2013;206(6):861–7.
45. Balch CM, Soong S-J, Thompson JF, et al. Age as a predictor of sentinel node metastasis among patients with localized melanoma: an inverse correlation of melanoma mortality and incidence of sentinel node metastasis among young and old patients. Ann Surg Oncol 2014;21(4):1075–81.
46. Cavanaugh-Hussey MW, Mu EW, Kang S, et al. Older age is associated with a higher incidence of melanoma death but a lower incidence of sentinel lymph node metastasis in the SEER databases (2003-2011). Ann Surg Oncol 2015; 22(7):2120–6.
47. Sinnamon AJ, Neuwirth MG, Yalamanchi P, et al. Association between patient age and lymph node positivity in thin melanoma. JAMA Dermatol 2017;153(9): 866–73.
48. Conic RRZ, Ko J, Damiani G, et al. Predictors of sentinel lymph node positivity in thin melanoma using the National Cancer Database. J Am Acad Dermatol 2019; 80(2):441–7.
49. Bartlett EK, Peters MG, Blair A, et al. Identification of patients with intermediate thickness melanoma at low risk for sentinel lymph node positivity. Ann Surg Oncol 2016;23(1):250–6.
50. Chang JM, Kosiorek HE, Dueck AC, et al. Stratifying SLN incidence in intermediate thickness melanoma patients. Am J Surg 2018;215(4):699–706.
51. Egger ME, Stevenson M, Bhutiani N, et al. Age and lymphovascular invasion accurately predict sentinel lymph node metastasis in T2 melanoma patients. Ann Surg Oncol 2019;26(12):3955–61.

52. Hanna AN, Sinnamon AJ, Roses RE, et al. Relationship between age and likelihood of lymph node metastases in patients with intermediate thickness melanoma (1.01-4.00 mm): A National Cancer Database study. J Am Acad Dermatol 2019;80(2):433–40.

53. Bello DM, Han G, Jackson L, et al. The prognostic significance of sentinel lymph node status for patients with thick melanoma. Ann Surg Oncol 2016;23(5):938–45.

54. Song Y, Azari FS, Metzger DA, et al. Practice patterns and prognostic value of sentinel lymph node biopsy for thick melanoma: a National Cancer Database study. Ann Surg Oncol 2019;26(13):4651–62.

55. Ferrone CR, Panageas KS, Busam K, et al. Multivariate prognostic model for patients with thick cutaneous melanoma: importance of sentinel lymph node status. Ann Surg Oncol 2002;9(7):637–45.

56. Gajdos C, Griffith KA, Wong SL, et al. Is there a benefit to sentinel lymph node biopsy in patients with T4 melanoma? Cancer 2009;115(24):5752–60.

57. Kachare SD, Singla P, Vohra NA, et al. Sentinel lymph node biopsy is prognostic but not therapeutic for thick melanoma. Surgery 2015;158(3):662–8.

58. Page AJ, Li A, Hestley A, et al. Increasing age is associated with worse prognostic factors and increased distant recurrences despite fewer sentinel lymph node positives in melanoma. Int J Surg Oncol 2012;2012:456987.

59. Balch CM, Soong S-J, Gershenwald JE, et al. Age as a prognostic factor in patients with localized melanoma and regional metastases. Ann Surg Oncol 2013;20(12):3961–8.

60. Fleming NH, Tian J, Vega-Saenz de Miera E, et al. Impact of age on the management of primary melanoma patients. Oncology 2013;85(3):173–81.

61. Richardson BS, Anderson WF, Barnholtz-Sloan JS, et al. The age-specific effect modification of male sex for ulcerated cutaneous melanoma. JAMA Dermatol 2014;150(5):522–5.

62. Ribero S, Davies JR, Requena C, et al. High nevus counts confer a favorable prognosis in melanoma patients. Int J Cancer 2015;137(7):1691–8.

63. Bataille V, Kato BS, Falchi M, et al. Nevus size and number are associated with telomere length and represent potential markers of a decreased senescence in vivo. Cancer Epidemiol Biomarkers Prev 2007;16(7):1499–502.

64. Kaur A, Ecker BL, Douglass SM, et al. Remodeling of the collagen matrix in aging skin promotes melanoma metastasis and affects immune cell motility. Cancer Discov 2019;9(1):64–81.

65. Ecker BL, Kaur A, Douglass SM, et al. Age-related changes in HAPLN1 increase lymphatic permeability and affect routes of melanoma metastasis. Cancer Discov 2019;9(1):82–95.

66. Cormier JN, Xing Y, Ding M, et al. Population-based assessment of surgical treatment trends for patients with melanoma in the era of sentinel lymph node biopsy. J Clin Oncol 2005;23(25):6054–62.

67. Wrightson WR, Wong SL, Edwards MJ, et al. Complications associated with sentinel lymph node biopsy for melanoma. Ann Surg Oncol 2003;10(6):676–80.

68. Moody JA, Ali RF, Carbone AC, et al. Complications of sentinel lymph node biopsy for melanoma - A systematic review of the literature. Eur J Surg Oncol 2017;43(2):270–7.

69. Koskivuo I, Hernberg M, Vihinen P, et al. Sentinel lymph node biopsy and survival in elderly patients with cutaneous melanoma. Br J Surg 2011;98(10):1400–7.

70. Sabel MS, Kozminski D, Griffith K, et al. Sentinel lymph node biopsy use among melanoma patients 75 years of age and older. Ann Surg Oncol 2015;22(7): 2112–9.
71. Chang CK, Jacobs IA, Vizgirda VM, et al. Melanoma in the elderly patient. Arch Surg 2003;138(10):1135–8.
72. Friedman CF, Wolchok JD. Checkpoint inhibition and melanoma: Considerations in treating the older adult. J Geriatr Oncol 2017;8(4):237–41.
73. Fulop T, Larbi A, Witkowski JM, et al. Immunosenescence and cancer. Crit Rev Oncog 2013;18(6):489–513.
74. Hodi FS, O'Day SJ, McDermott DF, et al. Improved survival with ipilimumab in patients with metastatic melanoma. N Engl J Med 2010;363(8):711–23.
75. Schachter J, Ribas A, Long GV, et al. Pembrolizumab versus ipilimumab for advanced melanoma: final overall survival results of a multicentre, randomised, open-label phase 3 study (KEYNOTE-006). Lancet 2017;390(10105):1853–62.
76. Weber J, Mandala M, Del Vecchio M, et al. Adjuvant nivolumab versus ipilimumab in resected stage III or IV melanoma. N Engl J Med 2017;377(19):1824–35.
77. Eggermont AM, Blank CU, Mandala M, et al. Adjuvant pembrolizumab versus placebo in resected stage III melanoma. N Engl J Med 2018;378(19):1789–801.
78. Kugel CH, Douglass SM, Webster MR, et al. Age correlates with response to anti-PD1, reflecting age-related differences in intratumoral effector and regulatory T-cell populations. Clin Cancer Res 2018;24(21):5347–56.
79. Perier-Muzet M, Gatt E, Peron J, et al. Association of immunotherapy with overall survival in elderly patients with melanoma. JAMA Dermatol 2018;154(1):82–7.
80. Jain V, Hwang WT, Venigalla S, et al. Association of age with efficacy of immunotherapy in metastatic melanoma. Oncologist 2019;24:1–5.

Management of Noncutaneous Melanomas

Ann Y. Lee, MD*, Russell S. Berman, MD

KEYWORDS

- Mucosal melanoma • Anorectal melanoma • Vulvovaginal melanoma
- Head and neck mucosal melanoma • Sinonasal melanoma

KEY POINTS

- Noncutaneous melanoma is associated with poor overall survival rates and high rates of metastatic disease.
- Mucosal melanomas are amelanotic in one-third to one-half of cases, which can cause difficulty in making the initial diagnosis.
- Elective nodal dissection is not recommended for mucosal melanoma. There is a paucity of data to support use of sentinel lymph node biopsy.
- Mucosal melanomas have overall higher rates of KIT mutations but much lower rates of BRAF mutations compared with cutaneous melanoma.

INTRODUCTION

Mucosal melanoma is a rare subtype of melanoma that represents only 1.3% of all melanoma cases[1] and has distinct clinical, biological, and management considerations compared with cutaneous melanoma. Unlike the dramatic and steady increase in the incidence of cutaneous melanoma, mucosal melanoma incidence rates have remained steady.[2] Furthermore, unlike cutaneous melanoma, there are no known risk factors for developing mucosal melanoma and there is no known association with sun exposure. However, most mucosal melanomas present with advanced-stage disease, possibly explained by the lack of early symptoms as well as the mucosal locations being less accessible to routine screening. Approximately one-third to one-half of patients with mucosal melanoma have nodal involvement at the time of presentation,[3,4] and the prognosis is generally very poor, with 5-year overall survival rates of approximately 25%.[3] Even for patients with localized disease, survival in patients with mucosal melanoma was significantly worse than for patients with

Department of Surgery, NYU Langone Health, 550 1st Avenue, NBV 15N1, New York, NY 10016, USA
* Corresponding author. 550 1st Ave., NBV 15N1, New York, NY 10016, USA
E-mail address: Ann.lee@nyulangone.org
Twitter: @AnnYLeeSurgOnc (A.Y.L.); @bermar01 (R.S.B.)

Surg Oncol Clin N Am 29 (2020) 387–400
https://doi.org/10.1016/j.soc.2020.02.004
1055-3207/20/© 2020 Elsevier Inc. All rights reserved.

cutaneous melanoma (10%–60% for various mucosal sites vs >90% for cutaneous),[2] suggesting a true difference in the biology of the two entities. The proximity of these tumors to other vital organs often makes local control challenging, and the rarity of this disease makes clinical trials, and even consistent data, difficult to achieve. Data and treatment options are often extrapolated from cutaneous melanoma, but it is not clear that this is appropriate.

Patients with mucosal melanoma tend to present in their 50s to 80s, with median age at presentation in the 60s (**Table 1**). Mucosal melanomas tend to occur near mucocutaneous junctions, with the most common sites being head and neck (55.4%), anorectal (23.8%), and vulvovaginal (18.0%).[3,5] Although mucosal melanoma has a slight female predominance with a female/male ratio of 1.85:1,[1] this is likely skewed by the frequency of vulvovaginal melanomas, which do not have a male counterpart. Different sites of mucosal melanoma have different incidence patterns by race and sex. Altieri and colleagues[4] performed a review of the population-based California Cancer Registry from 1988 to 2013 and found that, although mucosal melanoma only represented 1% of melanomas in non-Hispanic white people, it accounted for 15% of melanomas in Asian/Pacific Islanders, 9% of melanomas in non-Hispanic black people, and 4% of melanomas in Hispanic people. They also found that anorectal mucosal melanomas were most common in female Asian/Pacific Islanders, whereas head and neck mucosal melanomas were most common among Hispanic people and genitourinary mucosal melanomas were most common in non-Hispanic white people.

This article discusses clinicopathologic features, staging, and management of locoregional disease for the 3 most common sites: head and neck, anorectal, and vulvovaginal. Because there is a paucity of site-specific data regarding available systemic therapy, this is covered in a more global sense in relation to mutational analysis and systemic therapy for mucosal melanoma at the end of this article.

Ocular melanoma accounts for approximately 3.7% of melanoma cases[1] and also has a distinct pattern of management compared with either mucosal or cutaneous melanoma. The diagnosis and primary tumor management of ocular melanoma is highly specialized and typically performed by an ophthalmic oncologist and not by a general surgical oncologist. Therefore, its management is not discussed in this article. The exceptions to this are regional therapies for ocular melanoma liver metastases, which are reviewed in an article on regional therapies elsewhere in this issue.

HEAD AND NECK MUCOSAL MELANOMA
Clinical Features, Staging, and Prognosis

Head and neck mucosal melanomas most commonly occur in the sinonasal region (up to two-thirds) followed by the oral cavity.[2,6] The most common presenting symptoms for sinonasal melanoma are epistaxis and nasal obstruction.[7] Oral cavity mucosal melanomas are most often asymptomatic and detected by the patient or on oral examination. There are some reports of preceding oral melanosis,[8] but there is no clear evidence that this represents a premalignant state. Because approximately half of all head and neck mucosal melanomas are amelanotic,[9] the primary tumor is not always distinguishable on examination from other tumors of the head and neck. Confirmation with a panel of standard markers for melanoma such as S100, melan-A, tyrosinase, and/or HMB45 is helpful to confirm the diagnosis.[9] Oral cavity melanomas are more likely than sinonasal melanomas to present with cervical nodal involvement (25% vs 6%)[6] and clinicians should routinely examine all patients for the presence of cervical lymphadenopathy. Standard work-up should include a complete history and physical, including endoscopic examination plus computed tomography (CT) and/or

Table 1
Clinicopathologic features of the most common sites of mucosal melanoma versus cutaneous melanoma

	Cutaneous Melanoma	Head and Neck Melanoma	Anorectal Melanoma	Vulvovaginal Melanoma
Incidence (per million)[1]	153.5	0.7	0.4	1
Median Age at Diagnosis (y)	63	61	68–71	63
Male/Female Predilection	Slight male predominance	Slight male predominance for oral cavity	1.6-fold higher in women	Female predominance
Presence of Amelanosis (%)	1.8–8	50	29–71	27
Staging Systems Used	AJCC cutaneous melanoma	AJCC head and neck mucosal melanoma Ballantyne 3-tier staging	AJCC cutaneous melanoma Ballantyne 3-tier staging	AJCC cutaneous melanoma Ballantyne 3-tier staging FIGO (cervical)
5-y Overall Survival (%)	89	All 25 Sinonasal 38	17	Vulvar 20–54 Vaginal 10–32
Common Mutations				
BRAF (%)	41–52	3.5–8	10	0–26
c-KIT (%)	3	5–9.5	24–33	18–22
NRAS (%)	18–28	0–4.8 (30 in sinonasal)	19	4–12
Other (%)	—	—	NF1 (20)	—

Abbreviations: AJCC, American Joint Commission on Cancer; FIGO, International Federation of Gynecology and Obstetrics; NF1, neurofibromatosis type 1.

MRI with contrast to define the anatomy of the primary tumor. PET/CT and/or CT scan of the chest/abdomen/pelvis and brain MRI may be considered in more advanced cases.[10]

Head and neck mucosal melanomas are the only mucosal melanomas that are represented in the eighth edition of the American Joint Commission on Cancer (AJCC) staging manual (**Table 2**).[11] Because of the aggressiveness of these lesions, the lowest T category that can be assigned is T3, in which tumors are limited to the mucosa and immediately underlying soft tissue. T4a represents tumors that involve deep soft tissue, cartilage, bone, or overlying skin, and T4b represents tumors that involve brain, dura, lower cranial nerves (IX–XII), masticator space, carotid artery, prevertebral space, or mediastinal structures. The regional lymph node (N) and distant metastasis (M) categories are dichotomized into the presence or absence of regional nodal metastases or distant metastases, respectively. Although the T, N, and M categories remain defined and are prognostic,[12] in the eighth edition of the AJCC staging manual the overall prognostic stage grouping was eliminated. An alternative staging criteria, which are used in other mucosal melanomas, is the 3-tier Ballantyne staging, in which stage I represents clinically localized disease, stage II represents regional lymph node disease, and stage III represents distant disease[13] (**Table 3**). Overall 5-year survival is

Table 2
Tumor, node, metastasis definitions for head and neck mucosal melanoma

Category	Criteria
T (Primary Tumor)	
T3	Tumor limited to mucosa and immediately underlying soft tissue, regardless of thickness or greatest dimension; eg, polypoid nasal disease and pigmented or nonpigmented lesions of the oral cavity, pharynx, or larynx
T4a	Moderately advanced disease. Tumor involving deep soft tissue, cartilage, bone, or overlying skin
T4b	Very advanced disease. Tumor involving brain, dura, skull base, lower cranial nerves (IX, X, XI, XII), masticator space, carotid artery, prevertebral space, or mediastinal structures
N (Regional Lymph Node)	
NX	Regional lymph nodes cannot be assessed
N0	No regional lymph node metastases
N1	Regional lymph node metastases present
M (Distant Metastasis)	
M0	No distant metastasis
M1	Distant metastasis present
Prognostic stage grouping: There is currently no proposed prognostic stage grouping	

Adapted from Amin MB, American Joint Committee on Cancer., American Cancer Society. AJCC cancer staging manual. Eight edition / editor-in-chief, Mahul B. Amin, MD, FCAP ; editors, Stephen B. Edge, MD, FACS and 16 others ; Donna M. Gress, RHIT, CTR - Technical editor ; Laura R. Meyer, CAPM - Managing editor. ed. Chicago IL: American Joint Committee on Cancer, Springer; 2017.

poor, ranging from 25% to 38%.[14–16] In retrospective studies, older age, anatomic site in the nasopharynx and paranasal sinuses, and presence of distant metastatic disease have all been associated with worse prognosis.[6,14,15] Studies have been mixed as to whether primary tumor thickness is associated with survival, which may suggest that thickness in some instances just reflects extent of local tumor invasion. Similarly, nodal disease has not always been associated with survival. The primary cause of therapeutic failure is distant metastasis.[17]

Surgical Management

When feasible, the National Comprehensive Cancer Network (NCCN) guidelines recommend surgical excision of the primary site followed by adjuvant radiation for T4a and high-risk T3 disease.[10] Because major resections in the head and neck region can be very morbid and type of surgery has not been shown to correlate with rates of distant metastasis or death, there has been a move toward less aggressive resections and more endoscopic resections.[7,18] For general surgical oncologists, these cases

Table 3
Ballantyne 3-tier staging for mucosal melanoma

Stage	Description
I	Localized disease
II	Regional nodal disease
III	Distant metastatic disease

should be undertaken with surgeons who have sufficient head and neck experience as well as plastic surgeons to assist in reconstruction, when appropriate. Patients with documented T4b disease are not recommended to have surgery, but instead should get primary radiation and/or systemic therapy versus a clinical trial (preferred, if available).

Although sentinel lymph node biopsy is feasible and reported case series suggest that there may be prognostic value to performing sentinel lymph node biopsy,[19,20] because of the paucity of data it is not recommended as a routine part of surgical management or staging. For sinonasal melanoma, there is a lower incidence of lymph node metastases, and a large retrospective study from MD Anderson found that lymph node status was not a significant predictor of outcome.[21] Therefore, elective lymph node dissection for sinonasal melanoma is not recommended and therapeutic lymph node dissections should only be done in the setting of clinically positive lymph nodes. Because oral cavity melanoma is associated with higher rates of nodal metastases, the role of elective neck dissection is less clear. The most recent NCCN guidelines do include neck dissection in the management algorithm for oral cavity melanomas that are clinically node negative, but this is not based on prospective data.[10]

Radiation Therapy

Adjuvant radiation in head and neck mucosal melanoma can improve locoregional control[7,17,22–25] and is recommended in the NCCN guidelines for T4a and strongly considered for T3 lesions. However, it has not been shown to have any survival benefit.[7,22,25] Patients with locally advanced, unresectable disease are candidates for definitive radiation to the primary tumor and high-risk lymph node basins.[10,23]

ANORECTAL MUCOSAL MELANOMA
Clinical Features, Staging, and Prognosis

Anorectal melanoma accounts for approximately 0.4% to 1.1% of all melanoma cases.[26,27] According to a Surveillance, Epidemiology, and End Results (SEER) database study, the median age at presentation is 71 years and there is a 1.6-fold higher incidence in women than in men.[28] The transitional zone of the anal canal contains melanocytes, which increase from the dentate line to the anoderm. However, melanocytes have also been shown to be present above the dentate line in the colorectal zone,[29] and both anal-based and rectal-based mucosal melanomas have been described. Because many of these occur at the mucocutaneous border, it can sometimes be unclear whether anal melanomas are of cutaneous origin or mucosal origin. Common presenting symptoms include bleeding, pain, pruritus, and a mass.[26,30] Similar to head and neck mucosal melanomas, diagnosis can be delayed because of high rates of amelanosis (29%–71%)[30–32] and these lesions may be mistaken for other, more common, benign anorectal conditions such as hemorrhoids or rectal polyps. Immunohistochemistry staining with S100, HMB-45, and Mart-1/Melan-A is helpful in confirming the diagnosis.[33] Initial work-up should include digital rectal examination and anoscopy/endoscopy for evaluation of extent of local disease as well as either PET/CT or CT of the chest, abdomen, and pelvis to rule out distant metastatic disease. Addition of pelvic MRI (**Fig. 1**) can be useful in determining the extent of local invasion as well as regional nodal disease, and brain MRI can be considered in advanced cases to rule out brain metastases.

Unlike head and neck mucosal melanoma, there are no AJCC staging criteria for anorectal melanoma. Although there are no standard staging criteria, the 3-tier Ballantyne staging is often used when stage I represents clinically localized disease, stage II

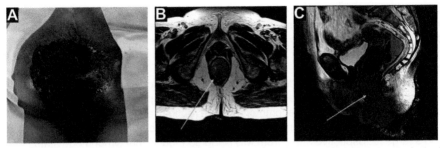

Fig. 1. Rectal melanoma with a long stalk and bulky disease extending past the anal canal on physical examination (*A*) and pelvic MRI (*B, C; arrows*).

represents regional lymph node disease, and stage III represents distant disease[13] (see **Table 3**). One study from MD Anderson studied 160 anorectal melanomas and found that the eighth edition AJCC cutaneous melanoma staging system was able to risk stratify patients with anorectal melanoma,[34] and is therefore used by some clinicians for staging. Primary tumor characteristics, including primary tumor thickness and lymphovascular invasion, correlated with disease-specific survival in patients with localized or regional disease but not with those who presented with distant metastases (with a universally poor prognosis). Up to a third of patients can present with metastatic disease[35] and overall 5-year survival is poor, ranging from 16% to 31%.[2,31,36,37] In retrospective studies, higher stage, presence of lymph node metastases, tumor thickness, amelanotic melanomas, and perineural invasion[26,34,36,38,39] have been associated with a worse prognosis.

Surgical Management

For patients with nonmetastatic disease, surgical excision remains the cornerstone of treatment. Historically, more aggressive surgical approaches, including abdominoperineal resection (APR) for anorectal melanoma, was the standard of care. However, many retrospective studies comparing the outcomes of APR with wide local excision have shown no difference in survival,[32,37,39] likely because there is a high rate of distant metastasis regardless of primary tumor surgical procedure. Therefore, if technically feasible, local excision with or without adjuvant radiation is preferred, with the ultimate goal of obtaining negative histologic margins (R0). In 1 retrospective study, R0 resection was associated with improved 5-year survival compared with patients with positive margins regardless of type of surgical approach (19% vs 6%, *P*<.001).[40] There have not been prospective trials investigating various clinical margins in mucosal melanoma. Use of at least a 1-cm margin with 1-cm to 2-cm margins for thicker lesions would be appropriate, although the risks and benefits of taking a larger margin must be carefully considered when additional margin is likely to result in additional morbidity. In particular, when assessing patients with bulky rectal melanomas, these can sometimes be attached to a smaller area of mucosa and extend with a stalk and therefore be amenable to local excision despite their bulky nature (see **Fig. 1**). The use of digital rectal examination, anoscopy/endoscopy, and MRI can be helpful in determining the best surgical approach. Although there is greater morbidity and additional quality-of-life issues associated with an APR, it still should be considered a treatment option for patients with localized bulky or recurrent disease.

The anorectal region has 2 potential lymphatic drainage patterns. Tumors can drain via the mesenteric nodes to the hypogastric and para-aortic nodes, or they can drain to the superficial inguinal lymph nodes. All potential draining nodal basins should be assessed by imaging and physical examination. Although there are case reports showing the technical feasibility of sentinel lymph node biopsy,[41–43] there is insufficient evidence to draw a conclusion about the prognostic or therapeutic value of the procedure, and there is currently no defined role for sentinel lymph node biopsy in anorectal melanoma. Given the variability in drainage patterns and high rates of distant metastasis, elective lymph node dissection is also not recommended. However, in the setting of clinically evident lymph node disease and in the absence of distant metastases, therapeutic lymph node dissection is recommended to gain regional control.

Radiation Therapy

Use of adjuvant radiation therapy in conjunction with sphincter-preserving local excision has been shown to be well tolerated and provide good local control but has not been associated with any improvement in overall survival.[36,44] Inclusion of inguinal nodal basins in the radiation field was not associated with improved outcome but did result in increased lymphedema.[44] Data are sparse on the use of primary radiation for treatment of anorectal melanoma. There are small case series in which patients do have temporary palliation of symptoms and it can be considered for selected patients with advanced disease or who are not surgical candidates.[45,46]

VULVOVAGINAL MUCOSAL MELANOMA
Clinical Features, Staging, and Prognosis

The 2 primary types of mucosal melanoma in the female genital tract are vulvar melanoma and vaginal melanoma. They both present with a median age in the 60s, but the range for vulvar melanomas is wider, with patients as young as 10 years old reported.[47] The most common presenting symptoms are pain, bleeding, pruritus, and/or a lesion/lump.[48,49] Approximately one-third of vulvovaginal melanomas are amelanotic and can be confused for other gynecologic lesions.[50,51] Dermoscopy may aid in differentiating melanoma from other pigmented vulvovaginal lesions.[52] Once biopsied, immunohistochemistry staining with a panel of S-100, HMB-45, Melan-A, tyrosinase, and MART-1 is helpful to confirm the diagnosis.[53] Standard work-up should include a pelvic examination and CT, MRI, and/or ultrasonography of the groin and pelvis to assess for locoregional disease (**Fig. 2**). In clinically suspected advanced cases, PET/CT and brain MRI may be used to rule out distant metastatic disease.

Similar to anorectal mucosal melanoma, there is no separate AJCC staging for vulvovaginal melanoma. The 3-tier Ballantyne staging used for other mucosal melanomas can be applied, in which stage I represents clinically localized disease, stage II represents regional lymph node disease, and stage III represents distant disease[13] (see **Table 3**). Previously, the AJCC staging for cutaneous melanoma has been applied to vulvar and vaginal melanomas and was shown to be prognostic.[54,55] Therefore, it is used by most treating physicians for vulvar and vaginal melanomas. In addition, some physicians have used the International Federation of Gynecology and Obstetrics (FIGO) 4-tier staging system used in other gynecologic malignancies, although this is primarily for cervical melanomas, which are very rare. Overall 5-year survival for vulvar melanomas ranges from 20% to 54%, and is worse for vaginal melanomas, approximately 10% to 32%.[50,56–59] Clinical features associated with worse prognosis include older age, regional nodal or distant disease, increased Breslow thickness, higher AJCC stage, and amelanosis.[47,49,54,60–62] Although the clitoral area and labia majora are the most common sites for vulvar melanoma,[63] centrally located vulvar lesions tend to be at higher risk of nodal involvement.[54]

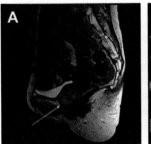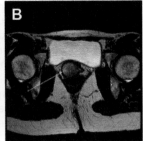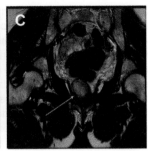

Fig. 2. (*A–C*) Pelvic MRI showing bulky vaginal melanoma (*arrows*) contained within the vaginal canal.

Surgical Management

Surgery is the cornerstone of treatment of primary vulvovaginal melanoma. Similar to anorectal melanoma, wide local excision and radical vulvectomy/pelvic exenteration have similar survival rates,[47,56,61] and therefore, when feasible, local excision is the preferred primary surgical treatment. There are no robust data regarding appropriate margins for local excision, but at least a 1-cm deep margin and 1-cm to 2-cm circumferential margin based on thickness and adjacent critical structures are generally recommended.[59,64]

Vaginal melanoma is similar to anorectal melanoma in its variable lymphatic drainage patterns, with drainage potentially to inguinal basins, pelvic basins, or both. There is a paucity of data regarding sentinel lymph node biopsy for vaginal melanomas and therefore no specific recommendations have been made.[59,64] In contrast with vaginal melanomas, sentinel lymph node biopsy for vulvar melanoma has been shown to be accurate and feasible, and it has been recommended by the Gynecologic Cancer Intergroup (GCIG) consensus review that patients with at least 1-mm thick vulvar melanomas undergoing wide local excision also be considered for a sentinel lymph node biopsy,[59,64,65] recognizing that there are few data compared with cutaneous melanoma. Elective lymph node dissection in patients with clinically negative regional nodal basins is not recommended. Regardless of primary site, patients with clinically positive lymph nodes without distant metastatic disease should undergo therapeutic lymph node dissection with the aim of improving locoregional control.

Radiation Therapy

Retrospective data have not shown any associated benefit of adjuvant radiation in vulvovaginal melanoma and it is therefore not routinely recommended.[47,58,64] A case series of 4 patients receiving ipilimumab with concurrent external beam radiation showed a favorable tumor response, with 1 having a complete pathologic response on pathologic review of the resection specimen.[66] Further studies combining radiation with checkpoint blockade are needed to validate these promising results.

MUTATIONAL ANALYSIS AND SYSTEMIC THERAPY FOR MUCOSAL MELANOMA

Because of the rarity of mucosal melanomas, there are few prospective studies for systemic therapy designed specifically for mucosal melanomas. Systemic therapy used in cutaneous melanoma has been extrapolated to use in mucosal melanoma, but generally with poor survival outcomes. Advanced cases of mucosal melanoma have been treated with cytotoxic chemotherapy in the past, but with a modest response rate to first-line therapy of about 10%.[67] A 3-arm phase II randomized trial of adjuvant high-dose interferon-α2b versus temozolomide plus cisplatin versus observation in Asian patients with resected mucosal melanoma showed that both regimens were safe and had better overall and recurrence-free survival compared with surgery alone.[68] Temozolomide plus cisplatin had longer median overall survival (48.7 vs 40.4 months) and longer median recurrence-free survival (20.8 months vs 9.4 months) compared with interferon. Exploratory subgroup analysis suggested that the benefit was mostly for head and neck mucosal melanomas.

More recently, attention has been drawn to potential use of targeted inhibitors and immunotherapy for mucosal melanoma. Overall, mucosal melanomas have a different genomic profile (see **Table 1**)[69–73] than cutaneous melanoma, which is associated with ultraviolet (UV) radiation exposure. As a whole, mucosal melanomas have an increased rate of c-KIT mutations (39%)[74] relative to cutaneous melanoma (~3%), but this is mostly caused by increased frequency in anorectal and vulvovaginal melanomas, not head and neck melanomas. For these patients, c-KIT inhibitors such as imatinib may be useful for patients with metastatic disease,[8,74–77] but development of imatinib resistance may limit the ability to have a durable response even in patients with imatinib-sensitive mutations.[78] Although BRAF mutations are fairly common in cutaneous melanoma (41%–52% of all cases, but higher in areas of chronic sun damage), they are rare in mucosal melanoma (~11% overall). In addition, many of the BRAF mutations documented are not the V600E mutation often seen in cutaneous melanoma.[79–81] However, patients with BRAF mutations may still respond to BRAF/MEK inhibitors, and should still be routinely included in the mutational analysis panel. NRAS mutations are overall less frequent in mucosal melanoma compared with cutaneous melanoma. However, among the mucosal melanomas, NRAS mutations have been shown to occur more frequently in anorectal[34] and sinonasal melanomas[82] and may be responsive to MEK inhibition, although the type of mutation alone has not been shown to have any prognostic value.

Some patients with mucosal melanoma were included in prospective randomized trials with immune checkpoint blockade. Retrospective review of the mucosal melanoma cohort treated in published prospective trials or as a part of an expanded access program found a 23% response rate to single-agent nivolumab or pembrolizumab, and 37% to combination ipilimumab with nivolumab.[83,84] However, progression-free survival was only 3 months and 6 months respectively, suggesting a continued need for effective systemic therapy for mucosal melanoma. A recent phase 1 clinical trial of an anti–programmed cell death protein 1 (PD-1) antibody (toripalimab) combined with an anti–vascular endothelial growth factor (VEGF) antibody (axitinib) found that, in an Asian population with metastatic mucosal melanoma, the combination was tolerable and resulted in objective responses in 14 of 29 (48%) chemotherapy-naive patients.[85] These data require validation in a larger cohort and with a non-Asian population as well.

SUMMARY

Mucosal melanoma is a rare disease with no identifiable risk factors. It has been difficult to standardize treatment of mucosal melanomas because of the rarity of the disease, a paucity of prospective data, and the lack of a uniformly accepted staging system. Overall prognosis is poor for all mucosal melanomas. Patients are more likely to present with advanced disease compared with cutaneous melanoma, which may be caused by lack of early symptoms and high rates of amelanosis (25%–70%) compared with cutaneous melanoma (1.8%–8%),[86,87] which adds to the difficulty in distinguishing melanoma from other more common, benign diseases.

Surgical management has moved toward wide local excision (when feasible) instead of more radical procedures. This shift in surgical approach is the result of the high likelihood of systemic failure regardless of extent of primary tumor surgery, and therefore no difference in overall survival outcomes based on type of surgery. Although therapeutic lymph node dissection for clinically evident disease is considered standard, there is a paucity of data regarding the utility of sentinel lymph node biopsy. Elective lymph node dissection has largely been abandoned.

Mutational analysis shows that mucosal melanomas differ from the usual UV radiation–associated changes seen in cutaneous melanoma, with mucosal melanomas having lower rates of BRAF mutation and higher rates of c-KIT mutations. Appropriate mutational analysis is important in advanced cases in which systemic therapy may be warranted. Although there is no clear best systemic therapy, the use of immunotherapy and/or targeted inhibitors shows some promise, and further clinical trials in this area will be of great interest to clinicians managing this disease.

DISCLOSURE

The authors have nothing to disclose.

REFERENCES

1. McLaughlin CC, Wu XC, Jemal A, et al. Incidence of noncutaneous melanomas in the U.S. Cancer 2005;103(5):1000–7.
2. Bishop KD, Olszewski AJ. Epidemiology and survival outcomes of ocular and mucosal melanomas: a population-based analysis. Int J Cancer 2014;134(12):2961–71.
3. Patrick RJ, Fenske NA, Messina JL. Primary mucosal melanoma. J Am Acad Dermatol 2007;56(5):828–34.
4. Altieri L, Wong MK, Peng DH, et al. Mucosal melanomas in the racially diverse population of California. J Am Acad Dermatol 2017;76(2):250–7.
5. Chang AE, Karnell LH, Menck HR. The National Cancer Data Base report on cutaneous and noncutaneous melanoma: a summary of 84,836 cases from the past decade. The American College of Surgeons Commission on Cancer and the American Cancer Society. Cancer 1998;83(8):1664–78.
6. Patel SG, Prasad ML, Escrig M, et al. Primary mucosal malignant melanoma of the head and neck. Head Neck 2002;24(3):247–57.
7. Moreno MA, Roberts DB, Kupferman ME, et al. Mucosal melanoma of the nose and paranasal sinuses, a contemporary experience from the M. D. Anderson Cancer Center. Cancer 2010;116(9):2215–23.
8. Seetharamu N, Ott PA, Pavlick AC. Mucosal melanomas: a case-based review of the literature. Oncologist 2010;15(7):772–81.
9. Williams MD. Update from the 4th edition of the World Health Organization classification of head and neck tumours: mucosal melanomas. Head Neck Pathol 2017;11(1):110–7.
10. NCCN clinical practice guidelines in oncology: head and neck cancers, version 3.2019. 2019. Available at: https://www.nccn.org/professionals/physician_gls/pdf/head-and-neck.pdf. Accessed September 17, 2019.
11. Amin MB, Edge S, Greene s, et al. In: AJCC cancer staging manual. 8th edition. Chicago: American Joint Committee on Cancer, Springer; 2017.
12. Koivunen P, Back L, Pukkila M, et al. Accuracy of the current TNM classification in predicting survival in patients with sinonasal mucosal melanoma. Laryngoscope 2012;122(8):1734–8.

13. Ballantyne AJ. Malignant melanoma of the skin of the head and neck. An analysis of 405 cases. Am J Surg 1970;120(4):425–31.

14. Jethanamest D, Vila PM, Sikora AG, et al. Predictors of survival in mucosal melanoma of the head and neck. Ann Surg Oncol 2011;18(10):2748–56.

15. Amit M, Tam S, Abdelmeguid AS, et al. Patterns of treatment failure in patients with sinonasal mucosal melanoma. Ann Surg Oncol 2018;25(6):1723–9.

16. Bachar G, Loh KS, O'Sullivan B, et al. Mucosal melanomas of the head and neck: experience of the Princess Margaret Hospital. Head Neck 2008;30(10):1325–31.

17. Liu ZP, Luo JW, Xu GZ, et al. Failure patterns and prognostic factors of patients with primary mucosal melanoma of the nasal cavity and paranasal sinuses. Acta Otolaryngol 2017;137(10):1115–20.

18. Hanna E, DeMonte F, Ibrahim S, et al. Endoscopic resection of sinonasal cancers with and without craniotomy: oncologic results. Arch Otolaryngol Head Neck Surg 2009;135(12):1219–24.

19. Prinzen T, Klein M, Hallermann C, et al. Primary head and neck mucosal melanoma: Predictors of survival and a case series on sentinel node biopsy. J Craniomaxillofac Surg 2019;47(9):1370–7.

20. Starek I, Koranda P, Benes P. Sentinel lymph node biopsy: A new perspective in head and neck mucosal melanoma? Melanoma Res 2006;16(5):423–7.

21. Amit M, Tam S, Abdelmeguid AS, et al. Approaches to regional lymph node metastasis in patients with head and neck mucosal melanoma. Cancer 2018; 124(3):514–20.

22. Li W, Yu Y, Wang H, et al. Evaluation of the prognostic impact of postoperative adjuvant radiotherapy on head and neck mucosal melanoma: a meta-analysis. BMC Cancer 2015;15:758.

23. Trotti A, Peters LJ. Role of radiotherapy in the primary management of mucosal melanoma of the head and neck. Semin Surg Oncol 1993;9(3):246–50.

24. Meleti M, Leemans CR, de Bree R, et al. Head and neck mucosal melanoma: experience with 42 patients, with emphasis on the role of postoperative radiotherapy. Head Neck 2008;30(12):1543–51.

25. Samstein RM, Carvajal RD, Postow MA, et al. Localized sinonasal mucosal melanoma: Outcomes and associations with stage, radiotherapy, and positron emission tomography response. Head Neck 2016;38(9):1310–7.

26. Wanebo HJ, Woodruff JM, Farr GH, et al. Anorectal melanoma. Cancer 1981; 47(7):1891–900.

27. DeMatos P, Tyler DS, Seigler HF. Malignant melanoma of the mucous membranes: a review of 119 cases. Ann Surg Oncol 1998;5(8):733–42.

28. Cote TR, Sobin LH. Primary melanomas of the esophagus and anorectum: epidemiologic comparison with melanoma of the skin. Melanoma Res 2009;19(1): 58–60.

29. Clemmensen OJ, Fenger C. Melanocytes in the anal canal epithelium. Histopathology 1991;18(3):237–41.

30. Chiu YS, Unni KK, Beart RW Jr. Malignant melanoma of the anorectum. Dis Colon Rectum 1980;23(2):122–4.

31. Brady MS, Kavolius JP, Quan SH. Anorectal melanoma. A 64-year experience at Memorial Sloan-Kettering Cancer Center. Dis Colon Rectum 1995;38(2):146–51.

32. Ward MW, Romano G, Nicholls RJ. The surgical treatment of anorectal malignant melanoma. Br J Surg 1986;73(1):68–9.

33. Balachandra B, Marcus V, Jass JR. Poorly differentiated tumours of the anal canal: a diagnostic strategy for the surgical pathologist. Histopathology 2007;50(1): 163–74.

34. Nagarajan P, Piao J, Ning J, et al. Prognostic model for patient survival in primary anorectal mucosal melanoma: stage at presentation determines relevance of histopathologic features. Mod Pathol 2020;33(3):496–513.
35. Thibault C, Sagar P, Nivatvongs S, et al. Anorectal melanoma–an incurable disease? Dis Colon Rectum 1997;40(6):661–8.
36. Ballo MT, Gershenwald JE, Zagars GK, et al. Sphincter-sparing local excision and adjuvant radiation for anal-rectal melanoma. J Clin Oncol 2002;20(23):4555–8.
37. Iddings DM, Fleisig AJ, Chen SL, et al. Practice patterns and outcomes for anorectal melanoma in the USA, reviewing three decades of treatment: is more extensive surgical resection beneficial in all patients? Ann Surg Oncol 2010; 17(1):40–4.
38. Pessaux P, Pocard M, Elias D, et al. Surgical management of primary anorectal melanoma. Br J Surg 2004;91(9):1183–7.
39. Yeh JJ, Shia J, Hwu WJ, et al. The role of abdominoperineal resection as surgical therapy for anorectal melanoma. Ann Surg 2006;244(6):1012–7.
40. Nilsson PJ, Ragnarsson-Olding BK. Importance of clear resection margins in anorectal malignant melanoma. Br J Surg 2010;97(1):98–103.
41. Sanli Y, Turkmen C, Kurul S, et al. Sentinel lymph node biopsy for the staging of anal melanoma: report of two cases. Ann Nucl Med 2006;20(9):629–31.
42. Olsha O, Mintz A, Gimon Z, et al. Anal melanoma in the era of sentinel lymph node mapping: a diagnostic and therapeutic challenge. Tech Coloproctol 2005; 9(1):60–2.
43. Damin DC, Rosito MA, Spiro BL. Long-term survival data on sentinel lymph node biopsy in anorectal melanoma. Tech Coloproctol 2010;14(4):367–8.
44. Kelly P, Zagars GK, Cormier JN, et al. Sphincter-sparing local excision and hypofractionated radiation therapy for anorectal melanoma: a 20-year experience. Cancer 2011;117(20):4747–55.
45. Harwood AR, Cummings BJ. Radiotherapy for mucosal melanomas. Int J Radiat Oncol Biol Phys 1982;8(7):1121–6.
46. Bujko K, Nowacki MP, Liszka-Dalecki P. Radiation therapy for anorectal melanoma–a report of three cases. Acta Oncol 1998;37(5):497–9.
47. Sugiyama VE, Chan JK, Shin JY, et al. Vulvar melanoma: a multivariable analysis of 644 patients. Obstet Gynecol 2007;110(2 Pt 1):296–301.
48. Wechter ME, Gruber SB, Haefner HK, et al. Vulvar melanoma: a report of 20 cases and review of the literature. J Am Acad Dermatol 2004;50(4):554–62.
49. Boer FL, Ten Eikelder MLG, Kapiteijn EH, et al. Vulvar malignant melanoma: Pathogenesis, clinical behaviour and management: Review of the literature. Cancer Treat Rev 2019;73:91–103.
50. Ragnarsson-Olding B, Johansson H, Rutqvist LE, et al. Malignant melanoma of the vulva and vagina. Trends in incidence, age distribution, and long-term survival among 245 consecutive cases in Sweden 1960-1984. Cancer 1993;71(5): 1893–7.
51. An J, Li B, Wu L, et al. Primary malignant amelanotic melanoma of the female genital tract: report of two cases and review of literature. Melanoma Res 2009; 19(4):267–70.
52. Murzaku EC, Penn LA, Hale CS, et al. Vulvar nevi, melanosis, and melanoma: an epidemiologic, clinical, and histopathologic review. J Am Acad Dermatol 2014; 71(6):1241–9.
53. Gupta D, Malpica A, Deavers MT, et al. Vaginal melanoma: a clinicopathologic and immunohistochemical study of 26 cases. Am J Surg Pathol 2002;26(11): 1450–7.

54. Phillips GL, Bundy BN, Okagaki T, et al. Malignant melanoma of the vulva treated by radical hemivulvectomy. A prospective study of the Gynecologic Oncology Group. Cancer 1994;73(10):2626–32.

55. Wechter ME, Reynolds RK, Haefner HK, et al. Vulvar melanoma: review of diagnosis, staging, and therapy. J Low Genit Tract Dis 2004;8(1):58–69.

56. DeMatos P, Tyler D, Seigler HF. Mucosal melanoma of the female genitalia: a clinicopathologic study of forty-three cases at Duke University Medical Center. Surgery 1998;124(1):38–48.

57. Pleunis N, Schuurman MS, Van Rossum MM, et al. Rare vulvar malignancies; incidence, treatment and survival in the Netherlands. Gynecol Oncol 2016;142(3): 440–5.

58. Kirschner AN, Kidd EA, Dewees T, et al. Treatment approach and outcomes of vaginal melanoma. Int J Gynecol Cancer 2013;23(8):1484–9.

59. Gadducci A, Carinelli S, Guerrieri ME, et al. Melanoma of the lower genital tract: Prognostic factors and treatment modalities. Gynecol Oncol 2018;150(1):180–9.

60. Ragnarsson-Olding BK, Nilsson BR, Kanter-Lewensohn LR, et al. Malignant melanoma of the vulva in a nationwide, 25-year study of 219 Swedish females: predictors of survival. Cancer 1999;86(7):1285–93.

61. Trimble EL, Lewis JL Jr, Williams LL, et al. Management of vulvar melanoma. Gynecol Oncol 1992;45(3):254–8.

62. Seifried S, Haydu LE, Quinn MJ, et al. Melanoma of the vulva and vagina: principles of staging and their relevance to management based on a clinicopathologic analysis of 85 cases. Ann Surg Oncol 2015;22(6):1959–66.

63. Ragnarsson-Olding BK, Kanter-Lewensohn LR, Lagerlof B, et al. Malignant melanoma of the vulva in a nationwide, 25-year study of 219 Swedish females: clinical observations and histopathologic features. Cancer 1999;86(7):1273–84.

64. Leitao MM Jr, Cheng X, Hamilton AL, et al. Gynecologic Cancer InterGroup (GCIG) consensus review for vulvovaginal melanomas. Int J Gynecol Cancer 2014;24(9 Suppl 3):S117–22.

65. Trifiro G, Travaini LL, Sanvito F, et al. Sentinel node detection by lymphoscintigraphy and sentinel lymph node biopsy in vulvar melanoma. Eur J Nucl Med Mol Imaging 2010;37(4):736–41.

66. Schiavone MB, Broach V, Shoushtari AN, et al. Combined immunotherapy and radiation for treatment of mucosal melanomas of the lower genital tract. Gynecol Oncol Rep 2016;16:42–6.

67. Shoushtari AN, Bluth MJ, Goldman DA, et al. Clinical features and response to systemic therapy in a historical cohort of advanced or unresectable mucosal melanoma. Melanoma Res 2017;27(1):57–64.

68. Lian B, Si L, Cui C, et al. Phase II randomized trial comparing high-dose IFN-alpha2b with temozolomide plus cisplatin as systemic adjuvant therapy for resected mucosal melanoma. Clin Cancer Res 2013;19(16):4488–98.

69. Lyu J, Wu Y, Li C, et al. Mutation scanning of BRAF, NRAS, KIT, and GNAQ/GNA11 in oral mucosal melanoma: a study of 57 cases. J Oral Pathol Med 2016;45(4):295–301.

70. Ozturk Sari S, Yilmaz I, Taskin OC, et al. BRAF, NRAS, KIT, TERT, GNAQ/GNA11 mutation profile analysis of head and neck mucosal melanomas: a study of 42 cases. Pathology 2017;49(1):55–61.

71. Yang HM, Hsiao SJ, Schaeffer DF, et al. Identification of recurrent mutational events in anorectal melanoma. Mod Pathol 2017;30(2):286–96.

72. Hou JY, Baptiste C, Hombalegowda RB, et al. Vulvar and vaginal melanoma: A unique subclass of mucosal melanoma based on a comprehensive molecular

analysis of 51 cases compared with 2253 cases of nongynecologic melanoma. Cancer 2017;123(8):1333–44.

73. Aulmann S, Sinn HP, Penzel R, et al. Comparison of molecular abnormalities in vulvar and vaginal melanomas. Mod Pathol 2014;27(10):1386–93.

74. Curtin JA, Busam K, Pinkel D, et al. Somatic activation of KIT in distinct subtypes of melanoma. J Clin Oncol 2006;24(26):4340–6.

75. Rivera RS, Nagatsuka H, Gunduz M, et al. C-kit protein expression correlated with activating mutations in KIT gene in oral mucosal melanoma. Virchows Arch 2008; 452(1):27–32.

76. Dumaz N, Andre J, Sadoux A, et al. Driver KIT mutations in melanoma cluster in four hotspots. Melanoma Res 2015;25(1):88–90.

77. Hodi FS, Corless CL, Giobbie-Hurder A, et al. Imatinib for melanomas harboring mutationally activated or amplified KIT arising on mucosal, acral, and chronically sun-damaged skin. J Clin Oncol 2013;31(26):3182–90.

78. Postow MA, Hamid O, Carvajal RD. Mucosal melanoma: pathogenesis, clinical behavior, and management. Curr Oncol Rep 2012;14(5):441–8.

79. Curtin JA, Fridlyand J, Kageshita T, et al. Distinct sets of genetic alterations in melanoma. N Engl J Med 2005;353(20):2135–47.

80. Lee JH, Choi JW, Kim YS. Frequencies of BRAF and NRAS mutations are different in histological types and sites of origin of cutaneous melanoma: a meta-analysis. Br J Dermatol 2011;164(4):776–84.

81. Cancer Genome Atlas Network. Genomic classification of cutaneous melanoma. Cell 2015;161(7):1681–96.

82. Amit M, Tam S, Abdelmeguid AS, et al. Mutation status among patients with sino-nasal mucosal melanoma and its impact on survival. Br J Cancer 2017;116(12): 1564–71.

83. Shoushtari AN, Munhoz RR, Kuk D, et al. The efficacy of anti-PD-1 agents in acral and mucosal melanoma. Cancer 2016;122(21):3354–62.

84. D'Angelo SP, Larkin J, Sosman JA, et al. Efficacy and safety of nivolumab alone or in combination with ipilimumab in patients with mucosal melanoma: a pooled analysis. J Clin Oncol 2017;35(2):226–35.

85. Sheng X, Yan X, Chi Z, et al. Axitinib in combination with toripalimab, a humanized immunoglobulin G4 monoclonal antibody against programmed cell death-1, in patients with metastatic mucosal melanoma: an open-label phase IB trial. J Clin Oncol 2019;37(32):2987–99.

86. Thomas NE, Kricker A, Waxweiler WT, et al. Comparison of clinicopathologic features and survival of histopathologically amelanotic and pigmented melanomas: a population-based study. JAMA Dermatol 2014;150(12):1306–14.

87. Koch SE, Lange JR. Amelanotic melanoma: the great masquerader. J Am Acad Dermatol 2000;42(5 Pt 1):731–4.

Sentinel Lymph Node Biopsy
Indications and Technique

Jessica Crystal, MD[a], Mark B. Faries, MD[b],*

KEYWORDS

- Melanoma • Sentinel lymph node • Metastasis • Staging

KEY POINTS

- Lymphatic mapping and sentinel lymph node biopsy are now standard components of treatment of intermediate-thickness melanomas (1–4 mm).
- Sentinel node status provides significant, independent staging information for patients with thick (>4 mm) melanomas.
- Sentinel lymph node biopsy provides staging information and is appropriate for selected patients with thin (<1 mm) melanomas.
- Proper performance of lymphatic mapping and sentinel lymph node biopsy requires participation or experienced clinicians in nuclear medicine, surgery, and pathology.
- Sentinel lymph node biopsy is therapeutic for regional control in most patients with regional metastases.

SENTINEL LYMPH NODE INDICATIONS
Historical Perspective

From the earliest reported clinical experience with melanoma, the importance of regional lymph node involvement has been recognized. The earliest case of melanoma reported in the English literature features a cervical lymph node metastasis in a patient with a melanoma of the face. Other similar experiences with lymphatic metastases influenced the understanding of metastasis in the disease and affected treatment recommendations including excision margins and the management of regional lymph nodes. One early treatise, delivered by the English surgeon Herbert Snow, recommended excision of regional lymph nodes immediately on diagnosis, even in the absence of clinically evident metastases.[1] He called this approach "anticipatory gland excision," which was subsequently referred to as elective lymph node dissection (ELND).

The hypothesis of ELND supporters was that regional lymph nodes functioned as filters or incubators for metastatic disease and that early removal of nodal metastases

[a] Cedars-Sinai Medical Center, 8700 Beverly Boulevard, Los Angeles, CA, USA; [b] The Angeles Clinic and Research Institute, Cedars-Sinai Medical Center, 11800 Wilshire Boulevard, Suite 300, Los Angeles, CA 90025, USA
* Corresponding author.
E-mail address: mfaries@theangelesclinic.org

Surg Oncol Clin N Am 29 (2020) 401–414
https://doi.org/10.1016/j.soc.2020.02.006
surgonc.theclinics.com

could interrupt a metastatic cascade and cure disease that would spread beyond the regional nodes if given time. Although experimental evidence has demonstrated that lymph nodes are not likely to be mechanical filters, their function as incubators of metastasis remains under active investigation. If this were true, ELND should improve survival in patients with melanoma. However, complete dissection of nodal basins is attended by the risk of some morbidity, leading to debate about whether the intervention was justifiable and eventually randomized clinical trials.

There were also efforts to determine which patients were candidates for early surgical intervention. Retrospective data suggested that patients with certain melanomas were more likely to benefit from surgery.[2] Patients with thin melanomas were felt to be at such low risk for both nodal and distant metastases that ELND was not warranted. Those with thick melanomas had relatively high risk for both nodal and distant disease and might not be saved by early surgery. It was the intermediate-thickness melanomas (variously defined, but often 1–4 mm) that had sufficient risk of nodal disease in the absence of distant metastases who would be most likely to benefit. Consequently, some of the randomized ELND trials focused on that population.

The ELND trials, overall, failed to show a significant survival advantage for early dissection, although most trials showed a trend in that direction, with significant benefit in some subgroups.[3–5] The debate that had started a century before might still be ongoing had sentinel lymph node (SLN) biopsy not been developed and reshaped the diagnostic and therapeutic landscape. The concept of a "sentinel" lymph node also has a long history, with several investigators suggesting specific locations of such a node for several types of tumors including cancers of the parotid and the penis.[6] However, current understanding of the SLN stems from an evolution of the ELND strategy.

In patients with primary melanomas in some locations, such as the trunk, determination of the most appropriate basin for an ELND was difficult due to variability in drainage. In the 1970s, Donald Morton and colleagues[7] evaluated lymphoscintigraphy as a means of determining the direction of lymphatic drainage. This proved to be a reliable way to identify which nodal basin was at risk. As radiotracers and imaging technology improved, it was apparent that specific lymph nodes could be seen as receiving drainage rather than an entire basin. Morton, Cochran and colleagues[8] began to explore removal of this dynamically defined lymph node as an indicator of the pathologic status of the entire basin. As initially reported in 1990, the SLN proved to be a highly reliable indicator, which quickly became a routine staging technique. Initially, completion lymph node dissection was recommended for all patients with metastases discovered in their SLNs.

Sentinel Lymph Node Impact on Staging

SLN biopsy has dramatically improved the accuracy of staging in melanoma due to the improved accuracy of pathologic evaluation possible with SLN relative to that performed on a full-dissection specimen. In the former, the pathologist is able to concentrate on a single or small number of nodes, allowing more sections to be evaluated and the use of immunohistochemical stains to enhance detection. Indeed, pathologic processing of SLN routinely identifies metastases with only small clusters or even individual melanoma cells.

What impact has that had on staging accuracy? The effect has been profound and repeatedly demonstrated. In one such study, Dessureault and colleagues[9] examined the outcomes of "node-negative" patients who had been staged using physical examination, ELND, or SLN biopsy. Survival among those who had only had nodal evaluation by physical examination was poor, approximately 69.8% at 5 years. Those who were deemed node negative by ELND did better but still had only a 77.7% survival at 5 years. It was only with SLN evaluation that patients could be accurately determined to be node negative, resulting in survival of 90.5% at 5 years in that group.

It is not unexpected then that when multivariable prognostic evaluations are done in the context of large retrospective datasets and in clinical trials SLN status typically is the most powerful determinant of outcome and is independent of other variables including thickness and ulceration.[10]

The most recent and perhaps strongest indicator of this effect can be seen in a comparison of the 2 most recent American Joint Committee on Cancer (AJCC) melanoma databases.[11] The database used in the seventh edition included patients who had either not been surgically staged or who had been evaluated using ELND as well as some who had SLN biopsy.[12] The eighth edition database required patients with melanomas T1b and above to have had SLN biopsy in order to be included. For the seventh edition, 5-year melanoma-specific survival for stage IIA, IIB, and IIC were 79% to 82%, 68% to 71%, and 53%. The same stages in the eight edition had survivals of 94%, 87%, and 82%,[11] which indicates a profound change in the accuracy of prognostication and confirming the essential nature of SLN biopsy. In the era of increasingly effective adjuvant therapy, this type of accurate staging is even more critical to optimal management.

Regional Disease Control

Uncontrolled regionally metastatic melanoma can be devastating, and achieving regional disease control is an important goal in itself. With the advent of SLN biopsy, the toxicity associated with achieving this goal became markedly reduced, as SLN biopsy is associated with markedly lower morbidity than ELND, and patients with negative SLN were spared that larger procedure.[13] The first Multicenter Selective Lymphadenectomy Trial (MSLT-I) demonstrated that nodal management with SLN biopsy followed by CLND among those with SLN metastases resulted in excellent long-term disease control in the regional nodal basin.[14] Similarly, the multicenter Sunbelt Melanoma Trial demonstrated low rates of regional nodal disease recurrence for patients managed in that way.[15] In addition, it seems that early dissection, guided by SLN biopsy, is associated with lower rates of lymphedema compared with later dissection in the presences of macroscopic disease.[16]

Perhaps even more significantly, it is becoming increasingly apparent that regional disease control can also be achieved in many cases by SLN biopsy alone. This is true because in most of the cases of SLN metastases, regional nodal disease is limited to the SLN.[17] In most patients who undergo CLND after SLN biopsy, no other nodal metastases are identified in the full dissection. Similarly, in the second MSLT study, three-quarters of patients with SLN metastases who did not undergo completion lymph node dissection were free of nodal recurrence in that basin over the long term **(Fig. 1)**.[18]

Survival

Perhaps the most controversial subject in regional management of melanoma is whether early nodal intervention improves survival. The answer may not be a simple yes or no. Earlier ELND trials did not show an overall benefit, as noted earlier. However, there seemed to be a consistent relationship of potential survival benefit with the thickness of the primary melanoma. Among thick melanomas (defined as >3.5 or >4 mm) there was no indication of benefit in any of the randomized trials.[4,10,19] Whereas, for intermediate thickness melanomas, there seemed to be a consistent signal of survival benefit, often to a significant degree, albeit in subgroup analyses.

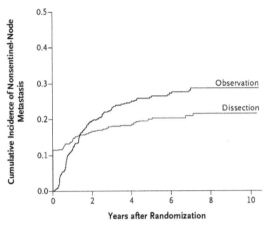

Fig. 1. Risk of in-basin nodal recurrence in the 2 arms of the second Multicenter Selective Lymphadenectomy Trial. All observation arm patients had had disease in SLN and had the remainder of their regional nodes left in place. Most do not demonstrate later recurrence in other regional nodes. (*From* Faries MB, Thompson JF, Cochran AJ, et al: Completion Dissection or Observation for Sentinel-Node Metastasis in Melanoma. N Engl J Med 376:2211-2222, 2017; with permission.)

MSLT-I was designed to evaluate the survival question as well and focused on an intermediate thickness (1.2–3.5 mm) group. In the final analysis, the number of events was lower than anticipated, making the trial underpowered, and the 3.1% increase in melanoma-specific survival seen in the SLN arm of the study was not significant ($P = .18$). However, examining the "node-positive" patients in the trial showed a marked difference in outcome (hazard ratio [HR] 0.56, 95% confidence interval [CI] 0.37–0.84, $P = .006$) for patients with nodal metastases removed with SLN-guided treatment compared with those with nodal recurrence in the observation arm. Given the risk of "ascertainment bias" with that simplistic analysis, a more statically sophisticated latent subgroup analysis was performed to try to adjust for any potential biases in the cohorts.[20,21] This also demonstrated a significant survival benefit associated with SLN management for the intermediate-thickness group but not the thicker primary patients. It is worth noting that although this statistical technique has been peer-reviewed and published in biostatistical journals, it is difficult to validate in other ways. Other retrospective series and meta-analyses also show a benefit. In the meta-analysis by Santos-Juanes and colleagues,[22] they found the melanoma-specific survival of SLN biopsy patients is better than that of wide local excision patients (HR 0.88, 95% CI 0.80–0.96).

So there remains a strong possibility that long-term survival is improved with early removal of nodal metastases and that this benefit depends on the thickness of the primary tumor. Other factors that may also play a role in the effectiveness of nodal treatment are primary tumor ulceration and patient age. However, the critical role of SLN biopsy in staging and regional control diminishes the relevance of the survival question in selecting patients for the procedure. It remains an important topic for translational research into the process of metastasis.

Selection for Sentinel Lymph Node Biopsy

The role of SLN biopsy in intermediate-thickness melanoma is now clear, and it is recommended for those patients in melanoma treatment guidelines of professional oncology organizations such as the American Society of Clinical Oncology, European Society of Medical Oncology, Society of Surgical Oncology, and national consensus panels in Australia, German, and Netherlands.[23–29] Other nonthickness factors such as age or potentially gene-expression profiling may further refine selection for SLN biopsy in this group, but at present it is a standard component of therapy. However, it is worth considering whether the same rationales can be applied in patients with thick (>4 mm) or thin (<1 mm) melanomas.

For thick melanomas, it has generally been felt that their prognosis is poor, even in the absence of nodal disease. However, numerous series now demonstrate that there is a significant association of long-term survival with the absence of nodal metastases on SLN biopsy.[30] This prognostic information may be of great importance with the increased variety of effective, although potentially toxic, adjuvant systemic therapies. In addition, it seems that even with thick primary melanomas, most patients with SLN metastases have no additional disease found on CLND, and the SLN biopsy may be therapeutic for regional control even in the absence of a full dissection.

Most of the patients with thin melanomas have no nodal metastases. Performance of the procedure for *all* such patients cannot be cost-effective or otherwise justified.[31] However, given the very large absolute number of patients with melanoma who present with thin primaries, the small proportion of node-positive patients in that population leads to substantial morbidity and mortality and identification of higher-risk patients with thin melanomas is an important goal.[32,33] In addition, the difference in survival between node-positive patients whose metastases were detected by SLN biopsy compared with those with clinical presentation of nodal recurrences is greatest in the thin melanoma population.[34] Although a randomized trial would not be feasible in this group, this comparison adds to the incentive to identify those at greatest risk for nodal disease.

The most widely applied factor for selection with thin melanomas is tumor thickness within the 0 to 1 mm range. The AJCC now divides T1a from T1b using a 0.8 mm cutoff.[35] Several guidelines, including American Society of Clinical Oncology/Society of Surgical Oncology and the National Comprehensive Cancer Network, recommend consideration of SLN biopsy for those with melanomas at least 0.8 mm in thickness.[28,29] Within that group, patient age, comorbidities, and other tumor factors including ulceration and mitotic rate may play a role in patient selection, although standard selection variables have not been consistently validated to firmly establish standards.

For melanomas thinner than 0.8 mm, the risk of nodal involvement is quite low, broadly observed to be less than 5%, and SLN biopsy is not routinely recommended for these patients. However, patients with "high-risk" characteristics in this group may be exceptions to that practice. Defining these high-risk features, again, has been challenging. Ulceration has frequently been found to be associated with nodal metastasis in these very thin lesions, although not in every series, and is rare in truly thin melanomas. Other features that have been considered include mitotic rate, Clark level of invasion, tumor-infiltrating lymphocytes, regression, and lymphovascular invasion, but there is marked inconsistency in which characteristics are useful across different series.[36,37] One final issue in selection is the deep margin of the biopsy. When a shallow shave biopsy is performed and tumor extends through the full depth of the evaluable material, the true depth of the lesion cannot be precisely determined. Some series have associated a positive deep margin with rates of nodal involvement similar to T1b or T2 melanomas.[38] Because a small additional area of tumor may have been ablated in the biopsy procedure or lost in a subsequent inflammatory response, even rebiopsy of the same area would not resolve the uncertainty. Examination of the biopsy slide will demonstrate the extent of margin involvement, which would also contribute to assessment of the nodal risk and recommendation for SLN biopsy.

The prognostic value of SLN staging in thin melanomas was a controversial issue early in the history of lymphatic mapping, but recent large series have now demonstrated fairly consistent findings.[39,40] Outcomes for patients with thin melanomas and SLN metastases are relatively favorable, although they are categorized as stage III. Melanoma recurrences and deaths in this group are relatively slow in appearing (few events before 2 years), but a modest decrease in survival has been consistently observed after that point. This is in contrast to the outcomes of patients with clinical nodal recurrences after local treatment of a thin primary melanoma, whose survival more closely approximates that of patients with macroscopic nodal metastases from intermediate or thick melanomas (stage IIIB/C).[34] Retrospective comparison of outcomes in patients with thin melanomas demonstrate much better survival for node-positive patients when metastases are discovered by SLN rather than recurrence, although ascertainment bias is a potential concern with such analyses.

SENTINEL LYMPH NODE PROCEDURE

Lymphatic mapping and SLN biopsy are simple in concept but require multidisciplinary expertise to be performed properly. Given the variable drainage patterns of primary melanoma sites, lymphoscintigraphy is essential to determine the location of SLNs.[41] Proper surgical technique is critical for identification, removal, and handling of the SLNs, and meticulous processing and pathologic evaluation is essential for both identification of metastases and assessment of their prognostic significance.

Lymphoscintigraphy and Ultrasound

In the early stages of the development of lymphatic mapping, lymphoscintigrams were performed to identify the draining nodal basins to direct ELNDs where multiple basins were at risk. Colloidal gold particles were used for this mapping, and imaging technology was somewhat rudimentary, with low-resolution images. As technology improved, it became apparent that lymphatic drainage could be traced not merely to the basin but to specific lymph nodes within the basin.

Radiopharmaceuticals used in lymphoscintigraphy vary in use around the world. In North America, sulfur colloid and tilmanocept are commonly used. Both are conjugated to ^{99m}technitium. Nanocolloid albumin is used in Europe and antimony trisulfide is used in Australia. Although there are potential functional differences in these agents, extensive experience in these different regions demonstrate that all can be used successfully.

Injection technique for the tracer is important for successful mapping. A narrow-gauge needle should be used to inject into the dermis surrounding the primary tumor site (ie, not subcutaneous). Often 4 peripheral injections are used, although the principle of injection is infiltration of lymphatic channels accessed by the primary tumor. With proper injection technique, massage of the area is generally unnecessary but may be performed to increase lymphatic flow.

Early dynamic images often identify and enumerate draining channels and document sequential or parallel drainage to SLNs. Imaging of all potential basins is also important, including minor basins such as the popliteal or epitrochlear locations in appropriate circumstances (**Fig. 2**).

In some circumstances, visualization of draining nodes by planar lymphoscintigraphy may be challenging, particularly when the primary tumor injection site is located close to or over the expected nodal location. In these instances, it is essential to

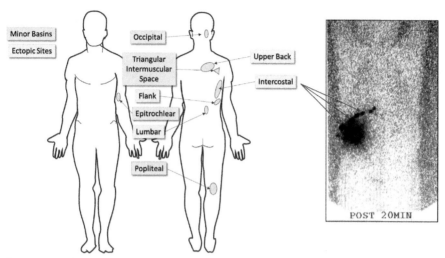

Fig. 2. Minor basins and ectopic SLN locations. Although SLNs are most often located in "standard" basin locations (cervical, axillary, inguinal) localization of SLNs outside of those areas is not uncommon. An example of intercostal SLNs is shown at right.

reevaluate the nodal basin intraoperatively with the gamma probe to verify removal of all SLNs. Three-dimensional imaging may also facilitate accurate identification of SLN in this and other complex settings. Single-photon emission computed tomography/computed tomography has been found to increase the number of detected SLNs and basins relative to planar lymphoscintigraphy alone.[42] It also provides more specific localizing information for SLNs, which may facilitate their identification and removal at the time of surgery.

Ultrasound seems to be the most sensitive modality for nodal evaluation before the biopsy procedure, frequently detecting disease before it is apparent on either physical examination or other imaging tests.[43–45] Suspicious nodal ultrasound characteristics include "rounding" of the node (length: width ratio <2), loss of hilar vascular echoes, thickening of the cortex, and particularly increased peripheral vascularity on Doppler imaging. The use of a high-frequency probe is necessary for accurate evaluations, and the experience of the operator is likely critical as well. However, even with optimal conditions, the sensitivity of ultrasound is low. The MSLT-II trial examined pre-SLN ultrasounds in its screening phase.[46] Ultrasound in this clinical context, at experienced melanoma centers, had a sensitivity of only 6.6%. Although this was higher in patients with thicker primary melanomas, the sensitivity never achieved a level that would enable observation of nodes that were negative by ultrasound. In addition, the principal rationale for pre-SLN ultrasound had been avoidance of SLN biopsy when the node was positive and proceeding directly with complete nodal dissection. Given the results of MSLT-II, this treatment pathway is no longer justified.

Operative Technique

The surgical portion of SLN biopsy must be completed with care and attention to detail to obtain the most accurate and least morbid results. The first step is confirmation of the draining basins. Review of the lymphoscintigram images and interrogation of the basins with the gamma probe before incision is important and allows appropriate adjustment in patient positioning if necessary (see **Fig. 2**). Planning of the SLN incision location should take the site of the primary tumor and reconstruction of that defect into account. In addition, the possible eventual need for a complete dissection should be considered, even though such dissections are becoming less common in current practice. In some locations, particularly the head and neck, understanding the likely location of nodes relative to surrounding structures may affect incision location to attempt to minimize dissection needed to reach the nodes.

Vital blue dye is injected before prepping the operative field. These dyes include lymphazurin, patent V, and methylene blue. Choice of dye is regional to some extent, with lymphazurin and methylene blue most commonly used in North America. Lymphazurin has been associated with allergic reactions, although these seem to be extremely uncommon in mapping for melanomas (relative to breast cancer).[13,47] Methylene blue has been associated with skin necrosis at the injection site, making it unacceptable if the entire injection site is not to be removed in the wide excision of the primary.[48] Similar to the technique for the tracer, using a small gauge needle vital blue dye is injected in small amounts around the primary lesion with care to inject the dermis (**Fig. 3**A, B).

Once an SLN has been identified using radiotracer and vital blue dye, dissection of the node requires considerable care. The node's capsule should not be grasped with forceps or clamps, as it is likely to tear (**Fig. 3**C, D). Because metastases are frequently located just beneath this capsule, its disruption may compromise the accuracy of the evaluation. The node may be pushed in the dissection and adjacent fibrous tissue may also be manipulated to isolate the node. Lymphatic channels entering the SLN can be controlled with clips or ligated, but all reasonable efforts should be made to preserve channels that are not entering the SLN.

Once the node has been removed, it should be examined again with the gamma probe to confirm its radioactivity. The surgeon may also consider marking the node at the site of highest activity or deepest blue staining, as this is likely to be the most

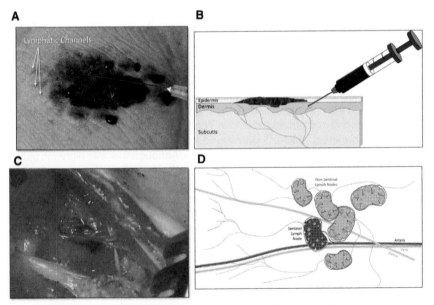

Fig. 3. (*A*) Injection of isosulfan blue should be intradermal and will often demonstrate peritumoral lymphatic channels. (*B*) Schematic of proper injection location, (*C*) View of SLN *in vivo* with undisturbed adjacent structures, (*D*) Schematic view of SLN *in vivo*.

common location of metastasis within the node, and communicating this with the pathologist. Surrounding lymph nodes within 10% of the highest tracer counts or with blue dye in them should also be excised.[15,49] Closure of the wound should include reapproximation of the lymphatic layer, while avoiding injury or entrapment of vessels or nerves in the process.

The decreased morbidity of SLN biopsy relative to complete dissection is one of the advantages of the technique, and efforts to minimize morbidity are essential, including preserving lymphatic tissue and vessels when possible. Although lymphedema is uncommon compared with CLND, it can occur. Injury or transection of motor or sensory nerves should be avoided. This is especially true in the head and neck region where the facial nerve is often close to parotid lymph nodes, the greater auricular nerve is often in the field of submandibular and jugulodigastric nodes, and the spinal accessory nerve is frequently close to nodes in Level V (**Fig. 4**).

Pathologic Processing

SLNs are sent for "permanent" pathologic evaluation. Frozen section should not be performed for several reasons.[50] First, the sensitivity of frozen section is substantially lower than with fixation, as small nodal metastases can be challenging to identify. In addition, freezing may introduce artifacts that make subsequent interpretation challenging and the tissue processing for frozen sections sacrifices potentially diagnostic material. Finally, because identification of an SLN metastasis no longer mandates immediate completion lymph node dissection, the main clinical rationale for rapid identification of nodal disease no longer exists.

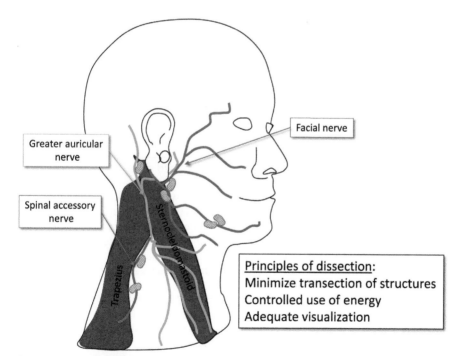

Fig. 4. SLNs are frequently located close to nerves. This is particularly true in the head and neck region. Care should be taken to avoid unnecessary transection of structures, indiscriminate use of energy devices, or operating through an incision that does not provide adequate visualization.

The SLN should be thoroughly sampled to ensure identification of metastases. Typically, nodes are bivalved along their long axis and the 2 faces placed in a single block. Sections are then obtained for staining with hematoxylin and eosin and immunohistochemical markers. These include combinations of S100, HMB45, Melan-A (MART-1), and Sox-10. Specific pathologic protocols vary around the world with regard to the exhaustiveness of sectioning and the specific stains used, but a combination of markers is recommended.

Pathologic Interpretation

Pathologic evaluation of the SLN provides the most valuable prognostic information for patients and clinicians, and an SLN free of metastasis indicates a much more favorable outlook for patients. However, the relative and absolute impact of SLN status varies to some extent for different patients and primary tumors. For example, older patients have a somewhat more guarded prognosis even in the absence of nodal metastases. This is particularly true for patients with thick or ulcerated primary tumors, who may have a substantial risk of recurrence. Adjuvant systemic therapies are currently being evaluated in those Stage II patients. At the other end of the spectrum, patients with SLN metastases from thin primary melanomas have a more favorable outlook. Melanoma recurrences in that group take longer (>2 years) to occur, and the long-term outlook is more favorable. However, for both thick and thin primary melanoma patients, SLN status provides independent and significant prognostic information.

Nodal tumor burden is also an important consideration in interpreting SLN results. Factors used to rate the seriousness of a metastasis include size, which is most commonly measured as the longest diameter of the largest metastatic focus, but which can also be measured by the absolute or relative area occupied by the metastasis. Other features include the number of metastatic foci, the penetrative depth into the node, and the location of the metastasis within the node (subcapsular, intraparenchymal, or both). The effect of tumor burden is likely a continuous variable with larger metastases being worse, but a cut off of 1 mm in most frequently used in maximal diameter.[51,52] This measure has been used for several retrospective analyses and as a cutoff for eligibility in clinical trials of adjuvant therapy.

Areas of Future Interest

Despite the extensive research that has been completed so far, there is more to be done. One area that needs to be further explored is in the immunobiology of the SLN. The SLN is the first organ encountered by tumor when traveling in the lymph system and first site where tumor antigens interact with the immune system. This subsequently plays an immunostimulatory role as it primes T cells specific to these tumor antigens. However, simultaneously, there is immunosuppressive interaction occurring in the SLN from immunosuppressive cytokines and regulatory T cells present. The complicated interaction of these 2 competing mechanisms is not fully defined and will be an important area of research into the future.[53,54]

There is also an interest in improving the technical aspects of SLN biopsy, which may improve the ease or accuracy of mapping. Examples include the use of fluorescent tracers, such as indocyanine green as a mapping agent with near-infrared detection techniques. These may be most helpful in the head and neck region, in which the target SLNs are relatively close to the surface (or in nonmelanoma cancers such as gastrointestinal malignancies).[55] These tracers also have the advantage of avoiding the use of radioactive tracers.[56] Another nonradioactive tracer is supermagnetic iron oxide.[57,58] These tracers are also detectable with MRI. The feasibility of their use has been demonstrated prospectively in breast cancer, with potential use in other malignancies including melanoma.

SUMMARY

SLN biopsy is now firmly established in the treatment of patients with melanoma, having documented irreplaceable benefits in staging and regional disease control. It should be routinely offered in intermediate and high-risk melanomas and considered in appropriately selected patients with thin melanomas. Additional refinements in our understanding of SLN biology and melanoma progression and in technical aspects of the procedure can be anticipated in coming years.

DISCLOSURE

M.B. Faries—Advisory Board: Novartis, Bristol Myers Squibb, Pulse Bioscience, Array Bioscience, Sanofi. Funding in part from NIH grant: 5R01CA189163.

REFERENCES

1. Neuhaus SJ, Clark MA, Thomas JM, et al. MRCS (1847-1930): the original champion of elective lymph node dissection in melanoma. Ann Surg Oncol 2004;11: 875–8.
2. Balch CM, Murad TM, Soong SJ, et al. Tumor thickness as a guide to surgical management of clinical stage I melanoma patients. Cancer 1979;43:883–8.
3. Veronesi U, Adamus J, Bandiera DC, et al. Delayed regional lymph node dissection in stage I melanoma of the skin of the lower extremities. Cancer 1982;49: 2420–30.
4. Cascinelli N, Morabito A, Santinami M, et al. Immediate or delayed dissection of regional nodes in patients with melanoma of the trunk: a randomised trial. WHO Melanoma Programme. Lancet 1998;351:793–6.
5. Balch C, Soong S, Ross M, et al. Long-term results of a multi-institutional randomized trial comparing prognostic factors and surgical results for intermediate thickness melanomas (1.0-4.0 mm). Ann Surg Oncol 2000;7:87–97.
6. Nieweg OE, Uren RF, Thompson JF. The history of sentinel lymph node biopsy. Cancer J 2015;21:3–6.
7. Holmes E, Moseley H, Morton D, et al. A rational approach to the surgical management of melanoma. Ann Surg 1977;186:481–90.
8. Morton D, Wen D, Wong J, et al. Technical details of intraoperative lymphatic mapping for early stage melanoma. Arch Surg 1992;127:392–9.
9. Dessureault S, Soong SJ, Ross MI, et al. Improved staging of node-negative patients with intermediate to thick melanomas (>1 mm) with the use of lymphatic mapping and sentinel lymph node biopsy. Ann Surg Oncol 2001;8:766–70.
10. Morton DL, Thompson JF, Cochran AJ, et al. Final trial report of sentinel-node biopsy versus nodal observation in melanoma. N Engl J Med 2014;370:599–609.
11. Gershenwald JE, Scolyer RA, Hess KR, et al. Melanoma staging: Evidence-based changes in the American Joint Committee on Cancer eighth edition cancer staging manual. CACancer J Clin 2017;67:472–92.
12. Balch CM, Gershenwald JE, Soong SJ, et al. Final version of 2009 AJCC melanoma staging and classification. J Clin Oncol 2009;27:6199–206.
13. Morton D, Cochran A, Thompson J, et al. Sentinel node biopsy for early-stage melanoma: accuracy and morbidity in MSLT-1, an interanational multicenter trial. Ann Surg 2005;242:302–11.

14. Morton DL, Thompson JF, Cochran AJ, et al. Sentinel-node biopsy or nodal observation in melanoma. N Engl J Med 2006;355:1307–17.
15. McMasters KM, Noyes RD, Reintgen DS, et al. Lessons learned from the sunbelt melanoma trial. J Surg Oncol 2004;86:212–23.
16. Faries MB, Thompson JF, Cochran A, et al. The impact on morbidity and length of stay of early versus delayed complete lymphadenectomy in melanoma: results of the Multicenter Selective Lymphadenectomy Trial (I). Ann Surg Oncol 2010;17: 3324–9.
17. Murali R, Desilva C, Thompson JF, et al. Non-Sentinel Node Risk Score (N-SNORE): a scoring system for accurately stratifying risk of non-sentinel node positivity in patients with cutaneous melanoma with positive sentinel lymph nodes. J Clin Oncol 2010;28:4441–9.
18. Faries MB, Thompson JF, Cochran AJ, et al. Completion dissection or observation for sentinel-node metastasis in melanoma. N Engl J Med 2017;376:2211–22.
19. Balch CM, Soong SJ, Smith T, et al. Long-term results of a prospective surgical trial comparing 2 cm vs. 4 cm excision margins for 740 patients with 1-4 mm melanomas. Ann Surg Oncol 2001;8:101–8.
20. Altstein LL, Li G, Elashoff RM. A method to estimate treatment efficacy among latent subgroups of a randomized clinical trial. Stat Med 2011;30:709–17.
21. Altstein L, Li G. Latent subgroup analysis of a randomized clinical trial through a semiparametric accelerated failure time mixture model. Biometrics 2013;69: 52–61.
22. Santos-Juanes J, Fernandez-Vega I, Galache Osuna C, et al. Sentinel lymph node biopsy plus wide local excision vs. wide location excision alone for primary cutaneous melanoma: a systematic review and meta-analysis. J Eur Acad Dermatol Venereol 2017;31:241–6.
23. Wong SL, Balch CM, Hurley P, et al. Sentinel lymph node biopsy for melanoma: American Society of Clinical Oncology and Society of Surgical Oncology joint clinical practice guideline. J Clin Oncol 2012;30:2912–8.
24. Dummer R, Guggenheim M, Arnold AW, et al. Updated Swiss guidelines for the treatment and follow-up of cutaneous melanoma. Swiss Med Wkly 2011;141: w13320.
25. Garbe C, Schadendorf D, Stolz W, et al. Short German guidelines: malignant melanoma. J Dtsch Dermatol Ges 2008;6(Suppl 1):S9–14.
26. Veerbeek L, Kruit WH, de Wilt J, et al. Revision of the national guideline "Melanoma". Ned Tijdschr Geneeskd 2013;157(12):A6136.
27. Dummer R, Hauschild A, Lindenblatt N, et al. Cutaneous melanoma: ESMO clinical practice guidelines for diagnosis, treatment and follow-up. Ann Oncol 2015; 26(Suppl 5):v126–32.
28. Wong SL, Faries MB, Kennedy EB, et al. Sentinel lymph node biopsy and management of regional lymph nodes in melanoma: American Society of Clinical Oncology and Society of Surgical Oncology Clinical practice guideline update. J Clin Onco 2018;36(4):399–413.
29. Coit DG, Thompson JA, Albertini MR, et al. Cutaneous melanoma, version 2.2019, NCCN clinical practice guidelines in oncology. J Natl Compr Canc Netw 2019;17: 367–402.
30. Rondelli F, Vedovati MC, Becattini C, et al. Prognostic role of sentinel node biopsy in patients with thick melanoma: a meta-analysis. J Eur Acad Dermatol Venereol 2012;26:560–5.
31. Agnese DM, Abdessalam SF, Burak WE Jr, et al. Cost-effectiveness of sentinel lymph node biopsy in thin melanomas. Surgery 2003;134:542–7 [discussion: 547–8].

32. Faries MB, Wanek LA, Elashoff D, et al. Predictors of occult nodal metastasis in patients with thin melanoma. Arch Surg 2010;145:137–42.

33. Karakousis GC, Gimotty PA, Botbyl JD, et al. Predictors of regional nodal disease in patients with thin melanomas. Ann Surg Oncol 2006;13:533–41.

34. Karakousis G, Gimotty PA, Bartlett EK, et al. Thin melanoma with nodal involvement: analysis of demographic, pathologic, and treatment factors with regard to prognosis. Ann Surg Oncol 2017;24:952–9.

35. Gershenwald JE, Scolyer RA, Hess KR. Melanoma of the skin. In: Amin MB, Edge SB, Greene FL, editors. AJCC cancer staging manual. New York: Springer International Publishing; 2017. p. 563–85.

36. Sondak VK, Messina JL, Zager JS. Selecting patients with thin melanoma for sentinel lymph node biopsy-this time it's personal. JAMA Dermatol 2017;153: 857–8.

37. Han D, Zager JS, Shyr Y, et al. Clinicopathologic predictors of sentinel lymph node metastasis in thin melanoma. J Clin Oncol 2013;31:4387–93.

38. Koshenkov VP, Shulkin D, Bustami R, et al. Role of sentinel lymphadenectomy in thin cutaneous melanomas with positive deep margins on initial biopsy. J Surg Oncol 2012;106:363–8.

39. Wright BE, Scheri RP, Ye X, et al. Importance of sentinel lymph node biopsy in patients with thin melanoma. Arch Surg 2008;143:892–9 [discussion: 899–900].

40. Mozzillo N, Pennacchioli E, Gandini S, et al. Sentinel node biopsy in thin and thick melanoma. Ann Surg Oncol 2013;20:2780–6.

41. Uren RF, Thompson JF, Howman-Giles R, et al. The role of lymphoscintigraphy in the detection of lymph node drainage in melanoma. Surg Oncol Clin N Am 2006; 15:285–300.

42. Vermeeren L, Valdes Olmos RA, Klop WM, et al. SPECT/CT for sentinel lymph node mapping in head and neck melanoma. Head Neck 2011;33:1–6.

43. Voit C, Mayer T, Kron M, et al. Efficacy of ultrasound B-scan compared with physical examination in follow-up of melanoma patients. Cancer 2001;91:2409–16.

44. Voit CA, van Akkooi AC, Eggermont AM. Role of ultrasound in the assessment of the sentinel node of melanoma patients. AJR Am J Roentgenol 2010;195:W474–5 [author reply: W476].

45. Starritt EC, Uren RF, Scolyer RA, et al. Ultrasound examination of sentinel nodes in the initial assessment of patients with primary cutaneous melanoma. Ann Surg Oncol 2005;12:18–23.

46. Thompson JF, Haydu LE, Uren RF, et al. Preoperative ultrasound assessment of regional lymph nodes in melanoma patients does not provide reliable nodal staging: results from a large multicenter trial. Ann Surg 2019. https://doi.org/10.1097/SLA.0000000000003405.

47. Liu Y, Truini C, Ariyan S. A randomized study comparing the effectiveness of methylene blue dye with lymphazurin blue dye in sentinel lymph node biopsy for the treatment of cutaneous melanoma. Ann Surg Oncol 2008;15:2412–7.

48. Neves RI, Reynolds BQ, Hazard SW, et al. Increased post-operative complications with methylene blue versus lymphazurin in sentinel lymph node biopsies for skin cancers. J Surg Oncol 2011;103:421–5.

49. Kroon HM, Lowe L, Wong S, et al. What is a sentinel node? Re-evaluating the 10% rule for sentinel lymph node biopsy in melanoma. J Surg Oncol 2007;95:623–8.

50. Cochran AJ, Huang R-R, Guo J, et al. Update on pathology evaluation of sentinel nodes from melanoma patients. In: Perry MC, editor. ASCO educational book. Alexandria (VA): American Society of Clinical Oncology; 2003. p. 1–5.

51. Egger ME, Bower MR, Czyszczon IA, et al. Comparison of sentinel lymph node micrometastatic tumor burden measurements in melanoma. J Am Coll Surg 2014;218:519–28.
52. Voit CA, van Akkooi AC, Schafer-Hesterberg G, et al. Rotterdam Criteria for sentinel node (SN) tumor burden and the accuracy of ultrasound (US)-guided fine-needle aspiration cytology (FNAC): can US-guided FNAC replace SN staging in patients with melanoma? J Clin Oncol 2009;27:4994–5000.
53. Cochran AJ, Huang RR, Lee J, et al. Tumour immunology - Tumour-induced immune modulation of sentinel lymph nodes. Nat Rev Immunol 2006;6:659–70.
54. Kim R, Emi M, Tanabe K, et al. Immunobiology of the sentinel lymph node and its potential role for antitumour immunity. Lancet Oncol 2006;7:1006–16.
55. Korn JM, Tellez-Diaz A, Bartz-Kurycki M, et al. Indocyanine green SPY elite-assisted sentinel lymph node biopsy in cutaneous melanoma. Plast Reconstr Surg 2014;133:914–22.
56. Vahabzadeh-Hagh AM, Blackwell KE, Abemayor E, et al. Sentinel lymph node biopsy in cutaneous melanoma of the head and neck using the indocyanine green SPY Elite system. Am J Otolaryngol 2018;39:485–8.
57. Douek M, Klaase J, Monypenny I, et al. Sentinel node biopsy using a magnetic tracer versus standard technique: the SentiMAG Multicentre Trial. Ann Surg Oncol 2014;21:1237–45.
58. Teshome M, Wei C, Hunt KK, et al. Use of a magnetic tracer for sentinel lymph node detection in early-stage breast cancer patients: a meta-analysis. Ann Surg Oncol 2016;23:1508–14.

Management of Regional Nodal Melanoma

Christina V. Angeles, MD[a], Sandra L. Wong, MD, MS[b],*

KEYWORDS

- Melanoma • Lymph nodes • Locoregional disease • Lymphadenectomy
- Nodal observation • Neoadjuvant/adjuvant therapy • Multidisciplinary care

KEY POINTS

- Complete nodal dissection is standard of care for clinically apparent nodal disease (with no evidence of distant metastases) along with consideration of adjuvant or neoadjuvant systemic therapy or enrollment in a clinical trial.
- Two prospective, randomized controlled trials show no significant benefit to performing a completion lymph node dissection (CLND) in sentinel lymph node–positive melanoma patients.
- Observation with ultrasound and clinical examination is an acceptable management strategy for sentinel lymph node biopsy–positive melanoma patients after consideration of patient-specific risks and benefits of forgoing CLND.
- The management strategy for regional nodal melanoma is evolving as ongoing investigations are being done with neoadjuvant and adjuvant therapies.

INTRODUCTION

Melanoma is the fifth most common cancer in the United States and one of the few with an increasing incidence. In fact, the rate of new melanoma diagnoses has been rising an average of 1.4% each year.[1] Although melanoma has historically been primarily a surgically treated disease due to poor systemic treatment options, recent advances in treatment with effective immunotherapy and targeted therapies have led to improvements in survival.[2–7] Along with these advances, the management of regional nodal melanoma has changed substantially.

The key management of clinical stage I and II melanoma remains primarily surgical in nature, with wide excision and sentinel lymph node biopsy (SLNB) for T1b or greater melanomas.[8] Nodal status continues to be the most informative prognostic factor for patients with clinically localized melanoma[9] and level I evidence demonstrates

[a] Department of Surgery, University of Michigan, 1500 East Medical Center Drive, Ann Arbor, MI 48109, USA; [b] Department of Surgery, Dartmouth-Hitchcock Medical Center, One Medical Center Drive, Lebanon, NH 03766, USA
* Corresponding author.
E-mail address: sandra.l.wong@hitchcock.org

Surg Oncol Clin N Am 29 (2020) 415–431
https://doi.org/10.1016/j.soc.2020.02.007
1055-3207/20/© 2020 Elsevier Inc. All rights reserved.

improved recurrence-free survival with SLNB than with nodal observation alone (no SLNB).[10] Following a positive-SLNB, completion lymph node dissection (CLND) had been the standard recommendation, but practice started to change, favoring observation and expectant management even before the data from 2 pivotal, prospective multi-institutional randomized controlled trials (RCTs) comparing CLND with observation demonstrated no statistical difference in survival endpoints at 3 years.[11–14]

With the changing landscape of melanoma management, including recent encouraging clinical trial results for neoadjuvant and adjuvant therapies for stage III melanoma,[15–17] it is imperative to have a good understanding of when and why to use a surgical approach to lymph node management.

EXTENT OF DISEASE

Regional nodal disease may present in patients as clinically occult, microscopic disease in the setting of a positive-SLNB, or as macroscopic disease in the setting of clinically evident, palpable or radiographic-detected lymph node(s). Given the high risk of distant metastatic disease in these patients,[18] it is essential that a thorough staging workup be done to evaluate for stage IV disease before making treatment decisions. In patients whose disease is limited to the nodal basins, their management differs based on whether they have microscopic or macroscopic disease.

Microscopic Disease

Until recently, the standard of care for patients found to have a positive-SLNB had been CLND of the involved nodal basin. This was based on the knowledge that about 15% to 20% of patients who undergo CLND will have additional nonsentinel lymph node (NSLN) disease, which is associated with poorer prognosis.[19–22] However, the clinical benefit of CLND had been increasingly questioned and there was evidence that CLND had been avoided in a high proportion of patients.[14,23–27] A recent meta-analysis of published retrospective studies and 2 RCTs looked at outcomes of observation versus CLND in the SLNB-positive population. Following a systematic review of the literature, 11 retrospective studies and 2 RCTs were found to have acceptable quality for inclusion in a meta-analysis. This included data from 8778 patients, 5895 of whom underwent CLND and 2883 who did not. Using event data and both locoregional and distant recurrences, meta-analysis showed no significant recurrence benefit for CLND compared with observation (risk ratio 0.91, 0.79–1.05; I^2 = 54%) (Fig. 1).[28] Additionally, there was no statically significant difference in survival between the 2 groups (risk ratio 0.85, 0.71–1.02, I^2 = 59%).[28]

When evaluating nodal recurrence rates, a higher incidence is expected in patients who undergo observation compared with CLND due to the known NSLN positivity rate found at the time of completion dissection.[19–21] Indeed, this was seen in the Multicenter Selective Lymphadenectomy II (MSLT-II) RCT with a rate of nodal recurrence 69% lower in the dissection group than in the observation group (hazard ratio [HR] 0.31, 95% confidence interval [CI] 0.24–0.41; $P<.001$), and just reached statistical significance in recurrence-free survival (RFS) (68% ± 1.7% in the CLND group and 63% ± 1.7% in the observation group; P = .05) with a median follow-up of 3.5 years.[11] In the Dermatologic Cooperative Group – Selective Lymphadenectomy (DeCOG-SLT) RCT, regional nodal recurrence was seen in 10.8% of patients who underwent CLND and 16.3% of those who were observed (not reported to be statistically different). Yet, the 5-year RFS rate was similar at 59.9% and 60.9%, respectively (HR 1.01, 90% CI 0.80–1.28; P = .94) with a median follow-up of 6 years. Interestingly, the DeCOG-SLT data now show that there may be less prognostic

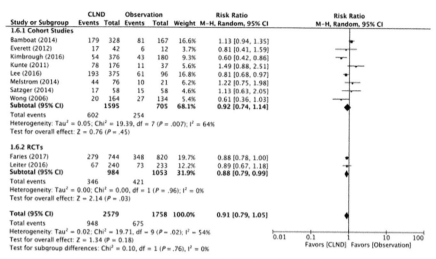

Study or Subgroup	CLND Events	CLND Total	Observation Events	Observation Total	Weight	Risk Ratio M-H, Random, 95% CI	Risk Ratio M-H, Random, 95% CI
1.6.1 Cohort Studies							
Bamboat (2014)	179	328	81	167	16.6%	1.13 [0.94, 1.35]	
Everett (2012)	17	42	6	12	3.7%	0.81 [0.41, 1.59]	
Kimbrough (2016)	54	376	43	180	9.3%	0.60 [0.42, 0.86]	
Kunte (2011)	78	176	11	37	5.6%	1.49 [0.88, 2.51]	
Lee (2016)	193	375	61	96	16.8%	0.81 [0.68, 0.97]	
Melstrom (2014)	44	76	10	21	6.2%	1.22 [0.75, 1.98]	
Satzger (2014)	17	58	15	58	4.6%	1.13 [0.63, 2.05]	
Wong (2006)	20	164	27	134	5.4%	0.61 [0.36, 1.03]	
Subtotal (95% CI)		**1595**		**705**	**68.1%**	**0.92 [0.74, 1.14]**	
Total events	602		254				
Heterogeneity: Tau² = 0.05; Chi² = 19.39, df = 7 (P = .007); I² = 64%							
Test for overall effect: Z = 0.76 (P = .45)							
1.6.2 RCTs							
Faries (2017)	279	744	348	820	19.7%	0.88 [0.78, 1.00]	
Leiter (2016)	67	240	73	233	12.2%	0.89 [0.67, 1.18]	
Subtotal (95% CI)		**984**		**1053**	**31.9%**	**0.88 [0.79, 0.99]**	
Total events	346		421				
Heterogeneity: Tau² = 0.00; Chi² = 0.00, df = 1 (P = .96); I² = 0%							
Test for overall effect: Z = 2.14 (P = .03)							
Total (95% CI)		**2579**		**1758**	**100.0%**	**0.91 [0.79, 1.05]**	
Total events	948		675				
Heterogeneity: Tau² = 0.02; Chi² = 19.71, df = 9 (P = .02); I² = 54%							
Test for overall effect: Z = 1.34 (P = 0.18)							
Test for subgroup differences: Chi² = 0.10, df = 1 (P = .76), I² = 0%							

Favors [CLND]   Favors [Observation]

Fig. 1. Meta-analysis of recurrence after completion lymph node dissection or observation of patients with sentinel lymph node-positive melanoma. (*From* Angeles CV, Kang R, Shirai K, et al: Meta-analysis of completion lymph node dissection in sentinel lymph node-positive melanoma. Br J Surg 2019;106:672-81.)

significance to NSLN status than previously thought.[13] Both RCTs showed no differences in overall survival.

Now that we have 2 RCTs that show no significant benefit to performing a CLND, SLNB-positive patients generally do not undergo immediate CLND. However, it is important for the surgeon to understand the patient demographics of those enrolled in these trials and the limitations of the studies. MSLT-II included patients with cutaneous melanoma of any site, of whom 18% had head and neck melanoma.[11] DeCOG-SLT only enrolled patients with truncal or extremity melanoma.[12] The median follow-up for MSLT-II and DeCOG-SLT was 3.5 years and 6.0 years, respectively. Most patients in both trials had only one positive sentinel lymph node (SLN) and a low volume of nodal metastases, with 66% of patients having <1 mm disease (**Table 1**). Therefore, the current data are limited by potentially underestimating the benefit of CLND in patients who have a larger tumor burden in the SLN. That said, CLND does not seem to influence the survival of those with higher tumor burden based on subgroup analyses. In the final analysis with 6-year median follow-up of DeCOG-SLT, the investigators performed a subgroup analysis of patients with ≤1 mm versus >1 mm SLN metastases and this distinction showed no effect of CLND on survival in either group.[13] In the MSLT-II trial, similar evaluation showed no difference as well.[11]

The question remains whether the patients who are ultimately found to have positive NSLN actually benefit from the immediate CLND. In the RCTs, only 16% to 18% of patients were found to have NSLN metastasis at the time of CLND. However, a much higher proportion of patients were found to have distant metastatic disease before or concurrent with local or regional recurrence, and therefore, CLND did not have a beneficial effect on total recurrence rates.[11–13] In addition, if a node-only recurrence is detected early (via close observation), as shown by both RCTs, delayed CLND provides the same survival benefit as immediate CLND.[11–13] Further study needs to be done to better prospectively identify a subset of SLNB-positive patients who may benefit from CLND.

Table 1
Select demographics and results of 2 randomized controlled trials comparing observation with completion lymph node dissection for patients with sentinel lymph node–positive melanoma

Characteristic	DeCOG-SLT[12,13]	MSLT-II[11]
# Patients, CLND/observation	240/233	744/820
Location of primary	Truncal and extremity only	Any site (18% head and neck)
Only 1 positive SLN	92%	81%
SLN micrometastasis ≤1 mm	66%	66%
Median follow-up, mo	72	43
Primary endpoint (CLND v OBS)	Distant metastasis-free survival (65% v 68%; $P = .87$)	Melanoma-specific survival (86% v 86%; $P = .42$)
Recurrence rate (CLND v OBS)	36% v 34%	38% v 42%

Abbreviations: CLND, completion lymph node dissection; DeCOG-SLT, Dermatologic Cooperative Group–Selective Lymphadenectomy; MSLT-II, Multicenter Selective Lymphadenectomy II; OBS, observation; SLN, sentinel lymph node.

What we do know is that completion node dissection gives us more thorough prognostic data. If a patient with a positive-SLNB, who has no evidence of additional disease on imaging, undergoes observation, then that patient likely will not be offered adjuvant therapy. However, if the same patient undergoes CLND and is found to have additional NSLN-positive disease, these data may lead to a recommendation of systemic therapy. Whether staging (and downstream decision making based on stage) are reasonable indications for performing a CLND continues to be debated.

Patients with a positive-SLNB should undergo a thorough discussion of their options and factors to consider when deciding between CLND and observation. This includes patient-specific clinicopathological findings that may increase the risk of additional disease (higher SLN tumor burden, head/neck primary, >2 mm thick primary melanoma, and number of SLNs involved),[29–32] the data from 2 RCTs showing no survival benefit of CLND, the morbidity of a lymph node dissection (discussed later in this article), the feasibility of observation, and patient preference (**Table 2**). The patients in both RCTs underwent rigorous surveillance with ultrasound and nodal examinations every 3 to 4 months for the first 2 years. This follow-up schedule must be discussed with the patient, and if not practical, one should consider CLND. Patients should also know that if nodal recurrence is detected with this observation schedule, delayed CLND is generally recommended given that the current data support CLND in the setting of lymph node–only recurrence. Nevertheless, there are several multidisciplinary discussions regarding the next phase of clinical trials, and neoadjuvant/adjuvant systemic therapy is increasingly being recommended. However, patients with stage IIIA disease have less than 20% risk of disease recurrence,[33] therefore observation without adjuvant therapy is generally recommended for this subset of patients.

The current data supporting the role of adjuvant therapy (immunotherapy and targeted therapies) for stage IIIB/C disease are based on trials that had required CLND for either SLNB-positive or clinically detected nodal disease (see section on Adjuvant Therapy, later in this article). This may be important when considering options with patients because eligibility criteria should be reviewed before treatment planning. Also, it is currently unknown what, if any, effect CLND had on the longer term endpoints of the trials.

Table 2
Advantages and disadvantages of completion nodal dissection versus observation in patients with sentinel lymph node (SLN)-positive melanoma

Nodal Strategy	Advantages	Disadvantages
Complete Lymph Node Dissection (CLND)	Therapeutic • Reduced risk of nodal relapse Prognostic • Non-SLN status is a predictor of survival • Complete nodal staging	Patient satisfaction • Reduced quality of life • Increased morbidity, including pain, wound complications, lymphedema
Observation	Therapeutic • Equivalent survival (even in the setting of relapse with delayed CLND) Patient satisfaction • ~85% of patients are spared CLND	Therapeutic • Risk of nodal relapse Prognostic • Lack of complete nodal staging Patient satisfaction • Expectation for surveillance (every 4 mo examinations and ultrasonography)

Macroscopic Disease

Patients who present with clinically detected nodal disease or a high nodal disease burden found at the time of SLNB have a worse prognosis, with 5-year survival ranging from 69% (stage IIIC) to 32% (stage IIID) (American Joint Commission on Cancer, Eighth Edition).[34] Any patient with a clinically suspicious node should undergo fine-needle aspiration (FNA) or core needle biopsy, with ultrasound guidance if needed, to confirm presence of melanoma to inform the next steps in management. FNA has been shown to have high sensitivity and specificity for identifying melanoma in enlarged lymph nodes.[35] If FNA or core biopsy is nondiagnostic, excisional biopsy may be performed, being mindful of incision placement because of possible conversion to therapeutic lymph node dissection (TLND). In addition, radiological staging (computed tomography [CT], PET/CT, MRI) should be done before any surgical intervention to rule out distant metastatic disease that would make TLND less beneficial.

The data supporting deferral of CLND in the setting of microscopic disease found on SLNB should not be generalized to the patients who present with clinically palpable nodal disease. Currently there are no data to support abandoning nodal dissection in the clinically node-positive patients and thus, TLND is still considered standard of care. Nevertheless, in this era of rapid discoveries of new immunotherapeutics and targeted agents, it would be disadvantageous for patients to not consider neoadjuvant and adjuvant approaches or enrollment to clinical trials, along with surgical intervention. Patients with clinically detected nodal disease have a 70% chance of relapse with surgery alone.[33,36]

In the setting of bulky nodal disease, a neoadjuvant approach has multiple potential benefits. If a patient responds to neoadjuvant therapy, the decrease in disease burden could potentiate a safer dissection along nerves and vessels. One could also gain knowledge about the responsiveness of the tumor to the particular therapy, which is not possible in the adjuvant setting. Evaluation of responsiveness also gives insight into the appropriate approach with adjuvant therapy. The neoadjuvant approach allows preoperative monitoring of response clinically and radiographically, and postoperative assessment of pathologic response. Also, many patients with bulky nodal disease may not have distant disease evident on imaging, yet they are high risk of harboring distant microscopic disease. These patients could benefit from systemic therapy sooner rather than later.

In patients harboring a susceptible *BRAF*-mutated tumor, one approach is using BRAF/MEK inhibitors upfront, which has a predictable, high response rate. BRAF/MEK inhibitor therapy also has an expected development of resistance in 6 to 9 months, therefore, planning surgery before this time may be essential. This approach may not only make lymph node dissection technically easier, but could improve RFS. A phase II randomized controlled trial in patients with high-risk, resectable stage III and IV BRAF-mutated melanoma showed improved event-free survival with 2 months of neoadjuvant and 10 months of adjuvant dabrafenib plus trametinib, compared with standard of care surgical resection followed by consideration of adjuvant interferon and/or radiation.[17]

A compelling theoretic benefit of using neoadjuvant immunotherapy lies in boosting one's immune system with checkpoint inhibitors while plenty of tumor antigen is present compared with the adjuvant setting when the tumor has been removed. In the neoadjuvant setting, more tumor antigens are ideally available to stimulate the immune system and prime a robust response. This was demonstrated in a randomized trial in which patients with locally/regionally advanced resectable melanoma were randomized to neoadjuvant ipilimumab 3 mg/kg or 10 mg/kg × 4 doses along with high-dose Inteferon-a2b (HDI), both of which were also administered following definitive surgery. Thirty-four percent of patients demonstrated a pathologic complete response (pCR). The tumor infiltrating lymphocytes (TIL) in the tumor microenvironment (TME) correlated with pCR, and the clonality of the TIL was found to be associated with improved relapse-free survival.[37] In addition, the tumor-associated clones in the blood correlated with amount of TILs and clonal diversity in the tumors, thereby demonstrating the influence of neoadjuvant systemic therapy on both the circulation and tumor microenvironment.

Recurrent Disease

In the setting of recurrent nodal disease, one should approach these patients similarly to the macroscopic, clinically node-positive patients. Nodal recurrence points toward a more aggressive biology with an increased risk of having additional distant disease[13,26] and extent of disease evaluation (re-staging) should be considered mandatory. If node-only recurrence is diagnosed, then CLND is reasonable, with consideration of adjuvant therapy due to the high risk of undetected distant micrometastatic disease. Another approach is neoadjuvant therapy for reasons discussed previously. This clinical scenario may become more frequent as practice changes away from CLND in this post MSLT-II and DeCOG-SLT era. Nevertheless, discussion at a multidisciplinary tumor board is recommended to consider these systemic options and clinical trials.

SURGICAL CONSIDERATIONS

CLND continues to be a necessary procedure in the surgical oncologist's armamentarium, albeit done less frequently in current practice. Patients with clinically apparent nodal disease, without any evidence of distant disease, have a 5-year survival of 30% to 50% after therapeutic lymphadenectomy[9,38,39] and there are no current data supporting better survival outcomes with nonsurgical therapy. Furthermore, there is still a role for palliative lymphadenectomy in the patient who is symptomatic and needs control of the regional nodal basin. A CLND entails a thorough dissection of the involved nodal basin, whether that basin was determined by a positive SLN or a clinically positive node.

There is some controversy over what defines an optimal nodal dissection. There are limited retrospective data that attempt to define the ideal number of lymph nodes that need to be removed for an adequate dissection,[40–43] and therefore, there are no agreed on guidelines, although there have been some threshold node counts proposed as minimum counts (used as proxies for the extent of dissection). To ensure high-quality care of the patient, the surgeon's operative note should include the anatomic boundaries of the dissection. Specifics of lymphadenectomy related to particular nodal basins are discussed as follows.

Cervical Lymphadenectomy

Melanoma located on the head and neck and the upper trunk can metastasize to the cervical lymph node basins. A modified neck dissection should be performed that includes levels II, III, IV, and V, and spares the spinal accessory nerve, the sternocleidomastoid muscle, and the internal jugular vein. If there are clinically positive or microscopically positive lymph nodes in the parotid gland, a superficial parotidectomy along with modified neck dissection on that side should be completed.[44] There has been discussion about doing a more selective node dissection with fewer anatomic regions in patients with only microscopic disease, yet there are no supporting data for this. Given the results of MSLT-II, observation of these patients is reasonable. If immediate CLND is elected, then a modified radical dissection should be performed. Patients who have disease with direct extension into a surrounding structure may require a radical neck dissection. According to expert opinion and retrospective data, the minimal number of nodes to be removed during a $\geq$4 level cervical neck dissection is 15 to 20 nodes.[40,41,45] However, the National Comprehensive Cancer Network (NCCN) guidelines do not recommend a specific number of nodes to be removed given the low level of supporting evidence.[46]

Axillary Lymphadenectomy

A complete axillary nodal dissection includes levels I, II, and III. This had been the standard of care for patients who were found to have axillary nodal disease. Now just as level III dissection was questioned for treatment of breast cancer (and current standard of care is dissection of levels I and II[47,48]), the utility in melanoma has been questioned. Level III disease is only found in 1.5% to 3.0% of patients with microscopic (positive-SLNB) axillary lymph node metastasis.[49,50] Many of these patients will not undergo CLND given the changing practice toward observation, and if they do elect CLND, it would be reasonable to dissect level III and remove any hard or enlarged nodes en bloc, or to complete a level III dissection if there is any concern for adenopathy on preoperative cross-sectional imaging. In a recent study, 17% of patients with clinically positive axillary lymph node melanoma metastases were found to have pathologic positive level III lymph nodes compared with 0% of SLNB-positive (microscopic disease) patients.[51] Therefore, CLND in these patients with recurrent disease should include levels I to III. Expert opinion suggests the minimum excised lymph nodes in a 3-level axillary lymphadenectomy should be at least 10 to 12.[40,41,45]

Inguinalfemoral (Superficial) and Ilioinguinal (Deep) Lymphadenectomy

In patients with microscopic positive-SLNB of the superficial inguinal nodal basin who elect CLND, an inguinalfemoral dissection is recommended. Many surgeons will excise the Cloquet node, which is the first deep pelvic node located under the inguinal ligament and posterior and medial to the external iliac vein. If the Cloquet node is found to be positive intraoperatively (clinically or frozen section), a deep dissection could be performed due to increased risk of positive deep lymph nodes. Over the past 10 to 15 years, most surgeons have shifted away from testing the Cloquet node in this setting based on data showing that the risk of having a positive pelvic lymph node is only 12%[52] and the difference in recurrence and survival of patients undergoing superficial versus superficial and deep dissections for SNLB-positive disease is not significant.[53,54] On the other hand, the risk of having pelvic nodal disease in the setting of palpable superficial inguinal nodal disease is 40% to 55%.[54,55] Current recommendation is to consider pelvic dissection in patients with suspicious iliac and/or obturator nodes on cross-sectional imaging (pelvic CT or PET/CT), palpable inguinalfemoral nodes, or ≥3 involved inguinal femoral nodes. These criteria all point to high-risk disease with poor survival, thereby bringing to question the benefit of doing a pelvic node dissection. In this evolving time with advances in systemic therapy, we may see more benefit with pelvic dissection than historical figures due to contemporary treatment planning with neoadjuvant or adjuvant therapy. Suggested minimum number of nodes to excise in a superficial (inguinal) dissection is 5 to 7, and in a superficial and deep (ilioinguinal) dissection, it is 13 to 14.[40,41,45,56]

Morbidity of Lymphadenectomy

When considering the option of lymphadenectomy as part of melanoma management, the risks and benefits need to be clearly discussed with the patient. Even before data from MSLT-II and DeCOG-SLT were available, only 50% of SLNB-positive patients actually underwent the previous standard of care CLND.[14] This is likely due to decision making based on the negative impact lymphadenectomy has on quality of life, which includes decreased mobility, pain, psychological distress, and chronic lymphedema.[11,57–59] On the other hand, the complications of bulky adenopathy should not be dismissed. Patients who present with late disease or who do not respond to systemic therapy may experience neuropathy, vascular congestion, compression of the airway (if in the cervical nodal basin), pain, and lymphedema. In these patients, the benefits of lymphadenectomy usually outweigh the risks; however, each patient's personal and disease characteristics will influence this balance. Both increased age and obesity have been shown to increase the complication rate.[60,61] Also, the severity of the morbidity is somewhat dependent on the specific nodal basin.

Modified radical neck dissection has a reported morbidity rate of approximately 10%.[62,63] The risks to the neurovascular structures are dependent on the extent of surgery and whether the parotid is involved. An even more selective approach to dissection has been considered to further reduce morbidities while maintaining similar recurrence and survival rates.[64]

Reported morbidity for axillary nodal dissection ranges from 20% to 50%.[62,63,65,66] Common complications include seroma, lymphocele, wound infection, axillary web syndrome (also known as cording), and loss of sensation due to injury to the intercostobrachial nerve. Chronic lymphedema is a major concern for patients, as it affects one's health-related quality of life.[59] In the breast cancer literature, postoperative lymphedema after axillary dissection has been reported as high as 13% to 50%,[67,68] yet rates appear to be much lower in the melanoma population (5%).[62,69]

Inguinal lymphadenectomy has a much higher incidence of overall morbidity and chronic lymphedema. This has been studied more thoroughly and multiple studies have shown overall morbidity of approximately 50% to 60% with complications including wound infection, wound dehiscence, prolonged seroma, skin flap necrosis, lymphedema, and deep vein thrombosis.[70,71] In the Sunbelt Melanoma Trial, 32% of patients who had an inguinal lymphadenectomy developed some lymphedema.[62]

To decrease this morbidity, other than considering alternatives to surgery (observation for SLN-positive disease and neoadjuvant systemic therapy for clinical positive disease), some techniques include preserving the saphenous vein, sparing the muscle fascia, sartorius transposition, and videoscopic minimally invasive techniques. Videoscopic inguinal lymphadenectomy has been shown to reduce wound complications while maintaining comparable oncological outcomes.[72]

ADJUVANT RADIATION

The use of adjuvant radiation (RT) for nodal disease could be considered in patients who are high risk for nodal relapse. The one prospective randomized trial (ANZMTG 01.02/TROG 02.01) that investigated adjuvant nodal RT versus observation after lymphadenectomy limited the trial to these high-risk patients, which they defined as any 1 of the following factors:

1. Involvement of ≥ 1 parotid nodes, ≥ 2 cervical or axillary nodes, or ≥ 3 inguinal nodes
2. Extranodal extension
3. Maximum diameter of the largest metastatic lymph node ≥ 3 cm for a cervical node or ≥ 4 cm for an axillary or inguinal node.[73,74]

The long-term data (median follow-up 73 months) showed a significant decrease in the risk of nodal relapse in the RT group (adjusted HR 0.52; 95% CI 0.31–0.88; $P = .023$), whereas there was no difference in overall survival or relapse-free survival (HR 1.27; 95% CI 0.89–1.79; $P = .21$, and HR 0.89; 0.65–1.22; $P = .51$, respectively.) Radiation does not come without side effects. In this study, 74% of patients experienced grade 2 to 4 toxic effects from radiotherapy (mostly pain and fibrosis of the skin or subcutaneous tissue) and 20% had grade 3 to 4 toxic effects. Limb assessments were performed over a period of 5 years and there was a significant increase in lower extremity lymphedema in the adjuvant radiotherapy group compared with observation (mean volume ratio 15.0% vs 7.7% [95% CI 1.5–13.1], $P = .014$). A nonsignificant difference was seen in the upper extremity (difference 3.4% [95% CI –3.0–9.3]; $P = .25$).

Notably, this trial was completed when the only adjuvant therapy available was interferon. Therefore, now that we have newer, more promising immunotherapies and targeted therapies, it is important to consider systemic therapy (which has a better chance to improve survival) as a first-line adjuvant therapy. The role of radiation therapy remains ill-defined despite the RCT data. Also, now that patients with melanoma have longer survival, the long-term effects of radiation may cause more harm than good.

ADJUVANT SYSTEMIC THERAPY

There is ongoing debate about which patients with regional nodal disease should or should not get adjuvant systemic therapy. Data from prospective trials with immune checkpoint inhibitor therapy show that there are consistently higher toxicity rates in the adjuvant compared with metastatic setting.[75,76] Therefore, one could speculate that waiting to treat with immunotherapy until there is a recurrence could result in an immune response to the tumor and less reactivity to self-antigens, or autoimmune side effects. Also, all of the stage III adjuvant trials to date have required CLND before adjuvant therapy, and now since MSLT-II and DeCOG-SLT, many of the positive-SLNB patients will not have a CLND but will be referred for adjuvant therapy. These practice changes are outside of the tested treatment protocols. Regional recurrences are increased in patients who do not have a CLND, yet if they do recur, they undergo salvage surgery and adjuvant therapy. Consequently, typical practice for stage IIIA patients with <1 mm tumor deposit in the SLNB is observation without adjuvant therapy. Patients with stage IIIA with ≥1 mm tumor deposit or IIIB/C will be referred for discussion of adjuvant therapy or clinical trial.

Ipilimumab (IPI), a CTLA-4 inhibitor, was the first new-age immunotherapy agent approved in the adjuvant setting. This was based on the results from the European Organization for Research and Treatment of Cancer (EORTC) 18,071 trial that evaluated high-dose IPI (10 mg/kg) versus observation in patients with high-risk, resectable stage III disease. There was improvement in overall survival (65.4% vs 54.4%) and RFS (26.1 vs 17.1 months) in the IPI group.[75] It is important, however, to note that many patients could not tolerate the high dose of IPI due to toxicity and more than half of the patients discontinued the drug, resulting in diminished enthusiasm for this adjuvant treatment.

The first PD-1 inhibitor approved in the adjuvant setting was nivolumab (NIVO). The CheckMate 238 trial evaluated high-dose IPI compared with NIVO in patients with resectable stage IIIB, IIIC, and IV melanoma. Patients who received NIVO had a significantly longer RFS than IPI at 1 year (71% vs 61%) and a lower rate of grade 3 or 4 adverse events (14% NIVO vs 46% IPI).[16] An update presented at the American Society of Surgical Oncology annual meeting in 2018 showed continued success with the 2-year RFS rates (63% NIVO vs 50% IPI.) No overall survival data are available, however, due to the superiority of NIVO along with its lower toxicity profile compared with IPI, oncologists prefer NIVO in the adjuvant setting.

Pembrolizumab (PEMBRO), a PD-1 inhibitor, was compared with placebo in the KEYNOTE-054/EORTC1345 study that looked at patients with completely resected stage III disease, including IIIA. PEMBRO was associated with a significantly longer RFS than placebo in the intention-to-treat group (75% vs 61%) and grade 3 or higher toxicities were found in 15% of patients.[76] Although it is too soon to have survival data, many patients and providers prefer PEMBRO in the adjuvant setting because of the every 3-week schedule compared with the every 2-week schedule for NIVO, and there is a lower toxicity profile compared with IPI.

Given that in 2 phase 3 trials (COMBI-d and COMBI-v) patients with unresectable or metastatic melanoma with *BRAF* V600E or V600K mutations had an improvement in overall survival with the BRAF inhibitor dabrafenib plus the MEK inhibitor trametinib,[5,77] this regimen was tested as an adjuvant therapy versus placebo for completely resected stage IIIA (lymph node metastases >1 mm), IIIB, or IIIC cutaneous melanoma in the COMBI-AD trial. Patients who received the combination therapy had an improved relapse-free survival and overall survival at 3 years (RFS: 58% combo vs 39% placebo, HR 0.47; 95% CI 0.39–0.58; $P<.001$, and overall survival: 86% combo vs 77% placebo, HR 0.57; 95% CI, 0.42–0.79; $P = .0006$).[15] It is recommended that all patients with stage III melanoma undergo BRAF tumor testing and for patients who have a BRAF mutation, oral dabrafenib/trametinib is a viable option in the adjuvant setting. As discussed previously, this is also a good option to use in the neoadjuvant setting for palpable or bulky nodal disease to decrease the extent of the surgical resection.

NEOADJUVANT TRIALS

To date there have been several small neoadjuvant systemic trials that included patients with clinical stage III melanoma. These trials had small sample sizes with various designs and endpoints, but all had early promising results with 19% to 58% pathologic complete response (pCR) rate and improved relapse-free survival.[17,37,78–82] Neoadjuvant dabrafenib plus trametinib followed by surgery and additional same adjuvant therapy has been shown to have 49% to 58% pCR and 20 to 23 months of relapse-

Table 3
Ongoing neoadjuvant clinical trials in stage III melanoma

Treatment Regimen	Patient Population	Phase	Study Outcomes	Trial Name Study ID
Neoadjuvant nivolumab ± ipilimumab or relatlimab and adjuvant nivolumab	Clinical stage III or oligometastatic stage IV	II	1° pathR 2° immunoR, objective response, RFS, OS, adverse effects	NCT02519322
Adjuvant vs neoadjuvant (plus adjuvant) pembrolizumab	Clinically detectable, resectable stage III-IV	II	1° Event-free survival 2° OS, disease control, pathR, RECIST, iRECIST	NCT03698019
Neoadjuvant and adjuvant dabrafenib and trametinib (single arm)	Resectable, clinical stage IIIB/C	II	1° RFS 2° OS, pCR, adverse events	Combi-Neo NCT02231775
Neoadjuvant dabrafenib, trametinib and/or pembrolizumab	BRAF V600 mutated resectable stage IIIB/C	II	1° PathR 2° RECIST, RFS, OS, postop complications, adverse events, operability, tumor/blood markers	NeoTrio NCT02858921
Neoadjuvant vemurarfenib, cobimetinib ± vemurafenib and atezolizumab	High-risk resectable stage III	II	1° pCR, RFS 2° Adverse events, change in PET/CT uptake	NeoACTIVATE NCT03554083
ipilimumab (3 or 10 mg/kg) and high-dose interferon α2b bracketing surgery	Resectable stage IIIB/C and IV	I	1° Adverse events 2° PathR, RadR, PFS, OS	NCT01608594[a]

Abbreviations: CT, computed tomography; immunoR, immunologic response; iRECIST, immune-related RECIST; OS, overall survival; PathR, pathologic response; pCR, pathologic complete response; PFS, progression free survival; RadR, radiological response; RECIST, response evaluation criteria in solid tumors; RFS, recurrence-free survival.

[a] Completed accrual, awaiting results.

free survival.[17,79] Also, there are encouraging early results from 2 trials of combination neoadjuvant checkpoint blockade with NIVO and IPI followed by adjuvant therapy with 45% to 57% pCR and greater than 80% relapse-free survival.[80,81] These and other results from early-phase trials have led to the current enthusiasm to investigate the clinical impact of neoadjuvant therapy in patients with clinical stage III melanoma.

There are multiple ongoing neoadjuvant melanoma trials for patients with resectable stage III melanoma, which are summarized in **Table 3**. These trials are investigating various immunotherapy and targeted therapeutic regimens and examining several clinical and pathologic outcomes, as well as adverse events. The neoadjuvant trial NCT01608594 looking at the combination of IPI and high-dose interferon α2b before and after surgery in resectable stage IIIB/C and IV melanoma has completed recruitment. The melanoma community eagerly awaits the results from these trials that are destined to be practice changing. Nonetheless, because many have both neoadjuvant and adjuvant in their design, deciding which approach is more beneficial will be challenging.

SUMMARY

The management of regional nodal melanoma has evolved and is continuing to evolve in an era of new discoveries and controversies. It is an exciting time with new data to support doing fewer lymph node dissections for microscopic nodal disease,[11,12] while creating a vigor to investigate which of these patients may actually benefit from dissection. At the same time, the extent of effective treatment options is expanding with both targeted and immunotherapies, affecting the decision making around the surgical management of melanoma, specifically related to the role of CLND.

For patients with microscopic, SLNB-positive melanoma (stage IIIA) with <1 mm of nodal disease, observation is recommended. For patients with SLNB-positive >1 mm nodal disease or stage IIIB, observation is reasonable as long as the patient understands the possibility of nodal relapse and later consideration of CLND. Patients with clinically evident nodal disease should be discussed at multidisciplinary tumor boards and be considered for neoadjuvant and/or adjuvant therapy and clinical trials; however, lymphadenectomy is still standard of care and should be performed. Salvage lymphadenectomy should be considered in patients who require regional control as long as the patient has been considered for systemic options and understands the risks and benefits of the procedure. The morbidity of lymphadenectomy is a significant factor in patient and surgeon decision making because of potential negative impacts on quality of life, including decreased mobility, pain, psychological distress, and chronic lymphedema, and therefore should always be discussed with the patient. The use of radiation should be limited to patients with high risk of nodal relapse who either failed systemic therapy or who are otherwise not candidates for systemic options as first-line adjuvant treatment given the increased morbidity without significant survival benefit.

There will continue to be evolution of the surgical management of nodal melanoma. Robust investigations are needed to inform continued high quality of care and improvement in outcomes for patients with melanoma.

DISCLOSURE

The authors have nothing to disclose.

REFERENCES

1. Anichini A, Maccalli C, Mortarini R, et al. Melanoma cells and normal melanocytes share antigens recognized by HLA-A2-restricted cytotoxic T cell clones from melanoma patients. J Exp Med 1993;177:989–98.

2. Hodi FS, O'Day SJ, McDermott DF, et al. Improved survival with ipilimumab in patients with metastatic melanoma. N Engl J Med 2010;363:711–23.

3. Robert C, Thomas L, Bondarenko I, et al. Ipilimumab plus dacarbazine for previously untreated metastatic melanoma. N Engl J Med 2011;364:2517–26.

4. Larkin J, Chiarion-Sileni V, Gonzalez R, et al. Combined nivolumab and ipilimumab or monotherapy in untreated melanoma. N Engl J Med 2015;373:23–34.

5. Robert C, Schachter J, Long GV, et al. Pembrolizumab versus ipilimumab in advanced melanoma. N Engl J Med 2015;372:2521–32.

6. Wolchok JD, Kluger H, Callahan MK, et al. Nivolumab plus ipilimumab in advanced melanoma. N Engl J Med 2013;369:122–33.

7. Postow MA, Chesney J, Pavlick AC, et al. Nivolumab and ipilimumab versus ipilimumab in untreated melanoma. N Engl J Med 2015;372:2006–17.

8. Wong SL, Faries MB, Kennedy EB, et al. Sentinel lymph node biopsy and management of regional lymph nodes in melanoma: American Society of Clinical Oncology and Society of Surgical Oncology Clinical Practice Guideline Update. J Clin Oncol 2018;36:399–413.

9. Balch CM, Soong SJ, Gershenwald JE, et al. Prognostic factors analysis of 17,600 melanoma patients: validation of the American Joint Committee on Cancer melanoma staging system. J Clin Oncol 2001;19:3622–34.

10. Morton DL, Thompson JF, Cochran AJ, et al. Final trial report of sentinel-node biopsy versus nodal observation in melanoma. N Engl J Med 2014;370:599–609.

11. Faries MB, Thompson JF, Cochran AJ, et al. Completion Dissection or Observation for Sentinel-Node Metastasis in Melanoma. N Engl J Med 2017;376:2211–22.

12. Leiter U, Stadler R, Mauch C, et al. Complete lymph node dissection versus no dissection in patients with sentinel lymph node biopsy positive melanoma (DeCOG-SLT): a multicentre, randomised, phase 3 trial. Lancet Oncol 2016;17:757–67.

13. Leiter U, Stadler R, Mauch C, et al. Final analysis of DeCOG-SLT Trial: no survival benefit for complete lymph node dissection in patients with melanoma with positive sentinel node. J Clin Oncol 2019;37(32):3000–8.

14. Bilimoria KY, Balch CM, Bentrem DJ, et al. Complete lymph node dissection for sentinel node-positive melanoma: assessment of practice patterns in the United States. Ann Surg Oncol 2008;15:1566–76.

15. Long GV, Hauschild A, Santinami M, et al. Adjuvant dabrafenib plus trametinib in stage III BRAF-mutated melanoma. N Engl J Med 2017;377:1813–23.

16. Weber J, Mandala M, Del Vecchio M, et al. Adjuvant nivolumab versus ipilimumab in resected stage III or IV melanoma. N Engl J Med 2017;377:1824–35.

17. Amaria RN, Prieto PA, Tetzlaff MT, et al. Neoadjuvant plus adjuvant dabrafenib and trametinib versus standard of care in patients with high-risk, surgically resectable melanoma: a single-centre, open-label, randomised, phase 2 trial. Lancet Oncol 2018;19:181–93.

18. Romano E, Scordo M, Dusza SW, et al. Site and timing of first relapse in stage III melanoma patients: implications for follow-up guidelines. J Clin Oncol 2010;28:3042–7.

19. Sabel MS, Griffith K, Sondak VK, et al. Predictors of nonsentinel lymph node positivity in patients with a positive sentinel node for melanoma. J Am Coll Surg 2005;201:37–47.

20. Lee JH, Essner R, Torisu-Itakura H, et al. Factors predictive of tumor-positive nonsentinel lymph nodes after tumor-positive sentinel lymph node dissection for melanoma. J Clin Oncol 2004;22:3677–84.

21. Morton DL, Cochran AJ, Thompson JF, et al. Sentinel node biopsy for early-stage melanoma: accuracy and morbidity in MSLT-I, an international multicenter trial. Ann Surg 2005;242:302–11 [discussion: 311–3].

22. Pasquali S, Mocellin S, Mozzillo N, et al. Nonsentinel lymph node status in patients with cutaneous melanoma: results from a multi-institution prognostic study. J Clin Oncol 2014;32:935–41.

23. Wong SL, Morton DL, Thompson JF, et al. Melanoma patients with positive sentinel nodes who did not undergo completion lymphadenectomy: a multi-institutional study. Ann Surg Oncol 2006;13:809–16.

24. Smith VA, Cunningham JE, Lentsch EJ. Completion node dissection in patients with sentinel node-positive melanoma of the head and neck. Otolaryngol Head Neck Surg 2012;146:591–9.

25. Mosquera C, Vora HS, Vohra N, et al. Population-based analysis of completion lymphadenectomy in intermediate-thickness melanoma. Ann Surg Oncol 2017; 24(1):127–34.

26. Bamboat ZM, Konstantinidis IT, Kuk D, et al. Observation after a positive sentinel lymph node biopsy in patients with melanoma. Ann Surg Oncol 2014;21:3117–23.

27. Satzger I, Meier A, Zapf A, et al. Is there a therapeutic benefit of complete lymph node dissection in melanoma patients with low tumor burden in the sentinel node? Melanoma Res 2014;24:454–61.

28. Angeles CV, Kang R, Shirai K, et al. Meta-analysis of completion lymph node dissection in sentinel lymph node-positive melanoma. Br J Surg 2019;106: 672–81.

29. Kibrite A, Milot H, Douville P, et al. Predictive factors for sentinel lymph nodes and non-sentinel lymph nodes metastatic involvement: a database study of 1,041 melanoma patients. Am J Surg 2016;211:89–94.

30. Gershenwald JE, Andtbacka RH, Prieto VG, et al. Microscopic tumor burden in sentinel lymph nodes predicts synchronous nonsentinel lymph node involvement in patients with melanoma. J Clin Oncol 2008;26:4296–303.

31. Murali R, Desilva C, Thompson JF, et al. Non-Sentinel Node Risk Score (N-SNORE): a scoring system for accurately stratifying risk of non-sentinel node positivity in patients with cutaneous melanoma with positive sentinel lymph nodes. J Clin Oncol 2010;28:4441–9.

32. Rossi CR, Mocellin S, Campana LG, et al. Prediction of non-sentinel node status in patients with melanoma and positive sentinel node biopsy: an italian melanoma intergroup (IMI) study. Ann Surg Oncol 2018;25:271–9.

33. Gershenwald JE, Scolyer RA, Hess KR, et al. Melanoma staging: evidence-based changes in the American Joint Committee on Cancer eighth edition cancer staging manual. CA Cancer J Clin 2017;67:472–92.

34. Gershenwald JE, Scolyer RA, Hess KR. Melanoma of the Skin. In: Amin MB, et al, editors. AJCC Cancer Staging Manual. 8th edition. Springer; 2017;47:563-585.

35. Hall BJ, Schmidt RL, Sharma RR, et al. Fine-needle aspiration cytology for the diagnosis of metastatic melanoma: systematic review and meta-analysis. Am J Clin Pathol 2013;140:635–42.

36. Balch CM, Gershenwald JE, Soong SJ, et al. Final version of 2009 AJCC melanoma staging and classification. J Clin Oncol 2009;27:6199–206.

37. Tarhini A, Lin Y, Lin H, et al. Neoadjuvant ipilimumab (3 mg/kg or 10 mg/kg) and high dose IFN-alpha2b in locally/regionally advanced melanoma: safety, efficacy and impact on T-cell repertoire. J Immunother Cancer 2018;6:112.

38. Spillane AJ, Pasquali S, Haydu LE, et al. Patterns of recurrence and survival after lymphadenectomy in melanoma patients: clarifying the effects of timing of surgery and lymph node tumor burden. Ann Surg Oncol 2014;21:292–9.

39. Khosrotehrani K, van der Ploeg AP, Siskind V, et al. Nomograms to predict recurrence and survival in stage IIIB and IIIC melanoma after therapeutic lymphadenectomy. Eur J Cancer 2014;50:1301–9.

40. Rossi CR, Mozzillo N, Maurichi A, et al. Number of excised lymph nodes as a quality assurance measure for lymphadenectomy in melanoma. JAMA Surg 2014;149:700–6.

41. Spillane AJ, Cheung BL, Stretch JR, et al. Proposed quality standards for regional lymph node dissections in patients with melanoma. Ann Surg 2009;249:473–80.

42. Xing Y, Badgwell BD, Ross MI, et al. Lymph node ratio predicts disease-specific survival in melanoma patients. Cancer 2009;115:2505–13.

43. Galliot-Repkat C, Cailliod R, Trost O, et al. The prognostic impact of the extent of lymph node dissection in patients with stage III melanoma. Eur J Surg Oncol 2006;32:790–4.

44. Pathak I, O'Brien CJ, Petersen-Schaeffer K, et al. Do nodal metastases from cutaneous melanoma of the head and neck follow a clinically predictable pattern? Head Neck 2001;23:785–90.

45. Bilimoria KY, Raval MV, Bentrem DJ, et al. National assessment of melanoma care using formally developed quality indicators. J Clin Oncol 2009;27:5445–51.

46. Coit DG, Thompson JA, Albertini MR, et al. Cutaneous melanoma, version 2.2019, NCCN clinical practice guidelines in oncology. J Natl Compr Canc Netw 2019;17:367–402.

47. Kiricuta CI, Tausch J. A mathematical model of axillary lymph node involvement based on 1446 complete axillary dissections in patients with breast carcinoma. Cancer 1992;69:2496–501.

48. Axelsson CK, Mouridsen HT, Zedeler K. Axillary dissection of level I and II lymph nodes is important in breast cancer classification. The Danish Breast Cancer Cooperative Group (DBCG). Eur J Cancer 1992;28A:1415–8.

49. Tsutsumida A, Takahashi A, Namikawa K, et al. Frequency of level II and III axillary nodes metastases in patients with positive sentinel lymph nodes in melanoma: a multi-institutional study in Japan. Int J Clin Oncol 2016;21:796–800.

50. Nessim C, Law C, McConnell Y, et al. How often do level III nodes bear melanoma metastases and does it affect patient outcomes? Ann Surg Oncol 2013;20:2056–64.

51. Mahvi DA, Fairweather M, Yoon CH, et al. Utility of level III axillary node dissection in melanoma patients with palpable axillary lymph node disease. Ann Surg Oncol 2019;26:2846–54.

52. Chu CK, Delman KA, Carlson GW, et al. Inguinopelvic lymphadenectomy following positive inguinal sentinel lymph node biopsy in melanoma: true frequency of synchronous pelvic metastases. Ann Surg Oncol 2011;18:3309–15.

53. Verver D, Madu MF, Oude Ophuis CMC, et al. Optimal extent of completion lymphadenectomy for patients with melanoma and a positive sentinel node in the groin. Br J Surg 2018;105:96–105.

54. Egger ME, Brown RE, Roach BA, et al. Addition of an iliac/obturator lymph node dissection does not improve nodal recurrence or survival in melanoma. J Am Coll Surg 2014;219:101–8.

55. Glover AR, Allan CP, Wilkinson MJ, et al. Outcomes of routine ilioinguinal lymph node dissection for palpable inguinal melanoma nodal metastasis. Br J Surg 2014;101:811–9.

56. Spillane AJ, Haydu L, McMillan W, et al. Quality assurance parameters and predictors of outcome for ilioinguinal and inguinal dissection in a contemporary melanoma patient population. Ann Surg Oncol 2011;18:2521–8.

57. Theodore JE, Frankel AJ, Thomas JM, et al. Assessment of morbidity following regional nodal dissection in the axilla and groin for metastatic melanoma. ANZ J Surg 2017;87:44–8.

58. Hyngstrom JR, Chiang YJ, Cromwell KD, et al. Prospective assessment of lymphedema incidence and lymphedema-associated symptoms following lymph node surgery for melanoma. Melanoma Res 2013;23:290–7.

59. Gjorup CA, Groenvold M, Hendel HW, et al. Health-related quality of life in melanoma patients: Impact of melanoma-related limb lymphoedema. Eur J Cancer 2017;85:122–32.

60. Friedman JF, Sunkara B, Jehnsen JS, et al. Risk factors associated with lymphedema after lymph node dissection in melanoma patients. Am J Surg 2015;210: 1178–84 [discussion: 1184].

61. Urist MM, Maddox WA, Kennedy JE, et al. Patient risk factors and surgical morbidity after regional lymphadenectomy in 204 melanoma patients. Cancer 1983;51:2152–6.

62. McMasters KM, Noyes RD, Reintgen DS, et al. Lessons learned from the sunbelt melanoma trial. J Surg Oncol 2004;86:212–23.

63. Guggenheim MM, Hug U, Jung FJ, et al. Morbidity and recurrence after completion lymph node dissection following sentinel lymph node biopsy in cutaneous malignant melanoma. Ann Surg 2008;247:687–93.

64. Geltzeiler M, Monroe M, Givi B, et al. Regional control of head and neck melanoma with selective neck dissection. JAMA Otolaryngol Head Neck Surg 2014; 140:1014–8.

65. van Akkooi AC, Bouwhuis MG, van Geel AN, et al. Morbidity and prognosis after therapeutic lymph node dissections for malignant melanoma. Eur J Surg Oncol 2007;33:102–8.

66. Karakousis CP, Hena MA, Emrich LJ, et al. Axillary node dissection in malignant melanoma: results and complications. Surgery 1990;108:10–7.

67. Lucci A, McCall LM, Beitsch PD, et al. Surgical complications associated with sentinel lymph node dissection (SLND) plus axillary lymph node dissection compared with SLND alone in the American College of Surgeons Oncology Group Trial Z0011. J Clin Oncol 2007;25:3657–63.

68. Taylor KO. Morbidity associated with axillary surgery for breast cancer. ANZ J Surg 2004;74:314–7.

69. Postlewait LM, Farley CR, Seamens AM, et al. Morbidity and outcomes following axillary lymphadenectomy for melanoma: weighing the risk of surgery in the era of MSLT-II. Ann Surg Oncol 2018;25:465–70.

70. Henderson MA, Gyorki D, Burmeister BH, et al. Inguinal and ilio-inguinal lymphadenectomy in management of palpable melanoma lymph node metastasis: a long-term prospective evaluation of morbidity and quality of life. Ann Surg Oncol 2019;26(13):4663–72.

71. Sabel MS, Griffith KA, Arora A, et al. Inguinal node dissection for melanoma in the era of sentinel lymph node biopsy. Surgery 2007;141:728–35.

72. Martin BM, Etra JW, Russell MC, et al. Oncologic outcomes of patients undergoing videoscopic inguinal lymphadenectomy for metastatic melanoma. J Am Coll Surg 2014;218:620–6.

73. Henderson MA, Burmeister BH, Ainslie J, et al. Adjuvant lymph-node field radiotherapy versus observation only in patients with melanoma at high risk of further

lymph-node field relapse after lymphadenectomy (ANZMTG 01.02/TROG 02.01): 6-year follow-up of a phase 3, randomised controlled trial. Lancet Oncol 2015;16: 1049–60.

74. Burmeister BH, Henderson MA, Ainslie J, et al. Adjuvant radiotherapy versus observation alone for patients at risk of lymph-node field relapse after therapeutic lymphadenectomy for melanoma: a randomised trial. Lancet Oncol 2012;13: 589–97.

75. Eggermont AM, Chiarion-Sileni V, Grob JJ, et al. Adjuvant ipilimumab versus placebo after complete resection of high-risk stage III melanoma (EORTC 18071): a randomised, double-blind, phase 3 trial. Lancet Oncol 2015;16:522–30.

76. Eggermont AMM, Blank CU, Mandala M, et al. Adjuvant pembrolizumab versus placebo in resected stage III melanoma. N Engl J Med 2018;378:1789–801.

77. Long GV, Stroyakovskiy D, Gogas H, et al. Combined BRAF and MEK inhibition versus BRAF inhibition alone in melanoma. N Engl J Med 2014;371:1877–88.

78. Amaria RN, Menzies AM, Burton EM, et al. Neoadjuvant systemic therapy in melanoma: recommendations of the International Neoadjuvant Melanoma Consortium. Lancet Oncol 2019;20:e378–89.

79. Long GV, Saw RPM, Lo S, et al. Neoadjuvant dabrafenib combined with trametinib for resectable, stage IIIB-C, BRAF(V600) mutation-positive melanoma (NeoCombi): a single-arm, open-label, single-centre, phase 2 trial. Lancet Oncol 2019;20:961–71.

80. Amaria RN, Reddy SM, Tawbi HA, et al. Neoadjuvant immune checkpoint blockade in high-risk resectable melanoma. Nat Med 2018;24:1649–54.

81. Rozeman EA, Menzies AM, van Akkooi ACJ, et al. Identification of the optimal combination dosing schedule of neoadjuvant ipilimumab plus nivolumab in macroscopic stage III melanoma (OpACIN-neo): a multicentre, phase 2, randomised, controlled trial. Lancet Oncol 2019;20:948–60.

82. Huang AC, Orlowski RJ, Xu X, et al. A single dose of neoadjuvant PD-1 blockade predicts clinical outcomes in resectable melanoma. Nat Med 2019;25:454–61.

Injectable Therapies for Regional Melanoma

Norma E. Farrow, MD[a], Margaret Leddy, PA-C, MMSc[b], Karenia Landa, MD[a], Georgia M. Beasley, MD, MHS[c],*

KEYWORDS

- In-transit melanoma • Intralesional therapies • Injectable therapies
- Melanoma vaccines • Immunotherapy • Oncolytic viral therapy

KEY POINTS

- Injectable therapies are a treatment option for patients with unresectable, recurrent, or refractory melanoma with cutaneous, subcutaneous, or nodal metastases.
- Advantages include ease of delivery to superficial disease sites, relatively limited systemic side-effect profile, and the ability to promote conversion of cold, noninflamed tumors to hot, immunologically engaged tumors.
- Injectable therapies include intralesional injection of oncolytic viruses, immune modulators, such as toll-like receptor agonists and inflammatory cytokines, gene therapy, and vaccines, among others.
- Talimogene laherparepvec, a modified oncolytic herpes virus, is the only Food and Drug Administration– approved injectable treatment currently in wide clinical use in the United States, with many more in development.
- In the future, injectable therapies will likely be most beneficial when used in conjunction with systemic therapies, such as immune checkpoint blockade.

INTRODUCTION

Although early-stage, localized melanoma is curable with surgical resection, a significant proportion of patients go on to develop recurrence. Approximately 4% to 12% of all patients develop recurrence in the form of in-transit (IT) disease, with involvement of dermal or subdermal lymphatics between the primary tumor site and the draining lymph nodes.[1,2] Patients with recurrent or metastatic disease, including IT

Research Support: N.E. Farrow and K. Landa receive research support from NIH-funded Surgical Oncology research training grant (T32 CA 93245). G.M. Beasley receives clinical trial funding from Istari Oncology.

a Department of Surgery, Duke University, Duke University Medical Center, Box 3443, Durham, NC 27710, USA; b Department of Surgery, Duke University, DUMC Box 3966, Durham, NC 27110, USA; c Department of Surgery, Duke University, DUMC Box 3118, Durham, NC 27710, USA
* Corresponding author.
E-mail address: georgia.beasley@duke.edu

Surg Oncol Clin N Am 29 (2020) 433–444
https://doi.org/10.1016/j.soc.2020.02.008
surgonc.theclinics.com

disease, have significantly decreased survival compared with those with localized disease.[1,3] Although patients with isolated locoregional disease may benefit from metastasectomies when it is possible to resect for curative intent, many of these patients develop multiple IT lesions that are unresectable and require alternative approaches. Patients with regional IT disease are classified by the American Joint Committee on Cancer (AJCC), 8th edition as having stage IIIB to IIID disease depending on the absence, presence, and extent of concurrent regional nodal involvement. Similar to IT locoregional disease, patients with stage IV M1a disease have one or more subcutaneous or dermal metastasis beyond the regional lymph node basin, and other patients with stage IV disease can also have concurrent subcutaneous disease.[4]

These cutaneous and subcutaneous tumor deposits pose a unique challenge for patients and providers, because they commonly become a source of discomfort, bleeding, and infection, and can be prohibitively morbid or impractical to resect. However, the superficial and accessible nature of these lesions provides the unique opportunity for treatment with intralesional therapy using injectable therapies, which are easy to deliver and generally have low-toxicity profiles. Intralesional therapies are thought to ideally work via local antitumor effects as well as the induction of tumor infiltrates and engagement of a systemic antitumor immune response. They have shown promise in select patients, leading to localized responses in the injected tumors and sometimes systemic or abscopal responses in distant lesions.[5,6]

Patients with IT or dermal metastases are eligible not only for injectable therapy but also for regional chemotherapy (limb only) and systemic therapy. Regional infusion therapies, indicated in a subset of patients with unresectable disease limited to an extremity, require general anesthesia and are limited by potentially severe limb toxicities.[7] Available systemic treatments now include multiple effective systemic therapies, including immune checkpoint blockade (ICB) and targeted therapy with BRAF/MEK inhibitors. Although these systemic therapies have shown remarkable gains in patient outcomes in recent years, they are limited by significant toxicity profiles and high costs of delivery as well as resistance to therapy and the development of recurrence.[8–10] Given the variety of treatment options currently available, the treatment strategy for advanced melanoma should be personalized and consider the number, location, and size of tumor deposits as well as the patient's condition and wishes. In addition, therapy should be multidisciplinary and is often multifactorial, using local, regional, and systemic therapies as well as surgical resection.

Numerous clinical trials are currently evaluating a variety of injectable therapies for advanced melanoma, including immune modulators, gene therapies, peptide vaccines, and oncolytic viruses, and the number of ongoing clinical trials investigating injectable therapies in melanoma has quickly surpassed the number of trials investigating limb infusion for locally advanced melanoma (**Table 1**). Intralesional therapy can be directly cytotoxic to tumors as well as promote tumor infiltration with immune cells, which has emerged as an important component of developing an antitumor response. Their role in the current landscape of treatment is evolving and includes the potential for therapeutic strategies combining injectable and systemic therapies, such as ICB, to convert and augment responses as well as use in the neoadjuvant or adjuvant settings.[11–14] This review covers the intralesional injectable therapies of historical importance, talimogene laherparepvec (T-VEC), which is the only currently Food and Drug Administration (FDA) - approved injectable therapy in wide clinical use, and promising therapies in development.

Table 1.
Number of total, completed (terminated, completed, and withdrawn), and active (not yet recruiting, recruiting, enrolling by invitation, and active, not recruiting) trials on clinicaltrials. gov in cutaneous melanoma when including search terms of virus, vaccine, and regional chemotherapy.

Search Term	Status	Number of Trials
Injectable/injection	Total	90
	Complete/active	55/32
Virus	Total	44
	Complete/active	23/19
Vaccine	Total	144
	Complete/active	113/44
Regional chemotherapy	Total	25
	Complete/active	19/4

Historical Agents

Bacille Calmette-Guérin

Bacille Calmette-Guérin (BCG) is a live-attenuated strain of *Mycobacterium bovis*, which has historically been used in the treatment of metastatic melanoma and other malignancies.[15,16] Intralesional injection of BCG produces a nonspecific inflammatory response and showed promise with reports of treatment responses in both injected and noninjected lesions, particularly cutaneous lesions (compared with subcutaneous lesions) and improvement in survival.[17] However, its use was associated with significant and sometimes severe side-effect profile, including malaise, flulike symptoms, hepatic dysfunction, and anaphylaxis.[18,19] Despite initial reports of high response rates, BCG failed to show a difference in disease-free or overall survival (OS) in stage I to III melanoma in a phase 3 randomized controlled trial and is now rarely used clinically.[20]

Interferon-α

Interferon-α (IFN-α) was used via systemic administration for patients with metastatic melanoma or in the adjuvant setting for many years, but was associated with significant toxicity and has now been largely replaced by newer therapies, such as ICB and targeted therapies.[21] It has also been used as an intralesional injection, although the evidence supporting its use is minimal and it is no longer used clinically.[22]

Interleukin-2

Another therapy used historically is interleukin-2 (IL-2), an endogenous immunomodulatory cytokine normally produced by activated T cells, which is important for T-cell survival and proliferation as well as augmentation of natural killer cell cytotoxicity.[23] IL-2 was initially used as intravenous systemic therapy, which showed a modest 10% to 15% response but was limited by high rates of toxicities.[24] Intralesional IL-2 was introduced in the 1980s and is generally well tolerated with common grade 1 to 2 adverse effects, including flulike symptoms and erythema but rare grade 3 to 4 toxicities, as well as promising response rate.[11,25] Although studies have not definitively shown an associated improvement in OS or noninjected lesions, a few studies have shown durable responses in a proportion of patients, with improvement in survival among complete responders.[11,26] More recent studies investigating IL-2 have explored recombinant forms of the cytokine as well as its use in conjunction with other systemic or local therapies.[13,27,28] One technique actively being investigated to improve the clinical benefit of intralesional IL-2 is through the combination of IL-2 with other cytokines and antibody fragments to promote delivery to and retention in the tumor. Daromun (L19-IL-2 + L19-tumor necrosis factor [TNF]) is a combination of the cytokines IL-2 and TNF each fused with the antibody fragment L19, which targets fibronectin expressed selectively in tumors.[13] Daromun has showed promise in a phase 2 trial, and a phase 3 trial is ongoing that will evaluate the added benefit of Daromun as neoadjuvant therapy in patients with stage IIIB/C melanoma undergoing surgery (NCT03567889). Outside of clinical trials, the use of IL-2 has decreased as more effective systemic therapies have been developed in recent years. In addition, its use remains limited because of the frequency of injections required as well as significant associated cost. However, like IFN and BCG, it remains an option for patients with unresectable disease when T-VEC is not available.[29]

Current and Developing Treatment Options

Oncolytic viral therapy

Talimogene laherparepvec Another treatment strategy in advanced melanoma is oncolytic viral therapy, or the use of viruses delivered directly to the tumor intralesionally, leading to direct cytotoxicity of tumor cells and the creation of an inflammatory response.[30] Talimogene laherparepvec (T-VEC; IMLYGIC) is an FDA-approved genetically modified type 1 herpes simplex viral immunotherapy developed to selectively infect and replicate in tumor cells. T-VEC causes direct cytolysis of tumor cells, recruits and activates immune cells, and drives production of granulocyte-macrophage colony-stimulating factor (GM-CSF), which stimulates the differentiation of progenitor cells into dendritic cells, maximizing the systemic immune response to the tumor.[31]

T-VEC was initially evaluated in a phase 1 trial in the early 2000s, in which 30 patients with cutaneous or subcutaneous tumor deposits of breast, head and neck, gastrointestinal, or refractory melanoma tumors received intratumoral injection of the virus.[32] The injections were generally well tolerated with the most common side effects being local inflammation, erythema, and febrile responses.[32] A subsequent phase 2 trial evaluating T-VEC in 50 patients with stage IIIC to IV melanoma revealed a 26% overall response rate (ORR) by RECIST (Response Evaluation Criteria in Solid Tumors) criteria, which showed responses not only in injected lesions but also in non-injected lesions, including visceral lesions.[33] This study found that adverse effects were limited primarily to transient flulike symptoms, which was consistent with the phase 1 trial.[33]

The OPTiM study was a phase 3 multicenter trial that enrolled 436 patients at 64 international sites with AJCC, 7th edition stage IIIB, IIIC, and IV unresectable melanoma with at least 1 injectable lesion and without bone metastases, active cerebral metastases, or visceral metastases greater than 3 cm or greater than 3 in number between 2009 and 2011. Most patients in each arm had stage IV disease, and about 47% of all patients had not yet had systemic therapy for melanoma. Patients were randomized in a 2:1 ratio to receive repeat intralesional injection with T-VEC or subcutaneous recombinant GM-CSF for a planned 6 months.[34] At a median treatment duration of 23 weeks in the T-VEC arm and 10 weeks in the GM-CSF arm, the study met its primary endpoint of durable response rate (DRR), defined as the rate of complete response (CR) or partial response lasting at least 6 months, noting a significantly higher DRR rate in the T-VEC arm of 16.3% versus the GM-CSF arm of 2.1% ($P<.001$). The ORR was also higher in the T-VEC arm (26.4% vs 5.7%), consistent with the phase 2 trial findings.[34] Median OS was 23.3 months in the T-VEC arm and 18.9 months in the GM-CSF arm ($P = .051$). The benefits of T-VEC were found to be more pronounced in patients with stage IIIB to IVM1a disease compared with those with later stage IV disease, with the improved DRR more pronounced in patients with stage IIIB or IIIC disease (33% vs 0%) and IVM1a disease (16% vs 2%) compared with patients with IVM1b (3% vs 4%). The results of the OPTiM trial ultimately led to FDA approval of T-VEC in 2015 as first-in-its-class oncolytic viral therapy, approved for intralesional (cutaneous, subcutaneous, and nodal lesions) treatment of unresectable stage III and stage IV melanoma.

In a recently published update, the OPTiM group presented an updated final analysis of the trial with a median follow-up of 49 months.[35] This updated analysis reports an improved DRR of 19.3% with T-VEC compared with 1.4% with GM-CSF, an ORR of 31.5% with T-VEC compared with 6.4% with GM-CSF.[35] Overall, 16.9% of patients in the T-VEC arm achieved a CR, with a median time to CR of 8.6 months, and achieving a CR was associated with improvement in OS. However, at this time, T-VEC has not been shown to improve survival when used as single therapy.[34,35] Similar to the primary OPTiM analysis, achieving a CR was significantly associated with earlier-stage metastatic disease (stage IIIB–IVM1a), as was DRR, ORR, and disease control rate. The T-VEC arm had an 11.3% grade 3 or 4 adverse event rate, including cellulitis (2.1%), fatigue, vomiting, dehydration, deep vein thrombosis, and tumor pain (each 1.7%). Although the most common adverse events seen with administration of T-VEC include fatigue, chills, pyrexia, nausea, and influenza-like illness, it is generally well tolerated and is currently in wide clinical use.

Oncolytic viruses, such as T-VEC, are thought to cause both specific and nonspecific inflammatory responses, leading to increased tumor immune infiltrates and creating an engaged immune microenvironment that may be better able to respond to systemic immune therapies, such as ICB or BRAF/MEK inhibitors.[30,36] Injectable therapies therefore have the potential to convert tumors that are devoid of immune cells ("cold" tumors) into tumors with immunologically engaged, T-cell–infiltrated microenvironments ("hot" tumors) that may be more responsive to systemic immune therapies. To this end, several recent and ongoing clinical trials (NCT02965716, NCT03972046) are investigating combinations of systemic therapies and T-VEC to enhance responses to systemic therapy.[36–39] In a phase 2 study of 198 patients with stage IIIB to IV unresectable melanoma comparing ipilimumab alone with combined ipilimumab with T-VEC, the combination therapy resulted in a significantly higher objective response rate (39% vs 18%, odds ratio, 2.9; 95% confidence interval, 1.5–5.5, $P = .002$), with responses in injected and noninjected lesions, including visceral lesions.[37] Adverse events grade 3 or higher were noted in 45% of patients in the combination group and 35% of the ipilimumab-alone group. Based on these results, this combination of intralesional T-VEC and ipilimumab is now considered a treatment option for certain patients with progression of metastatic or unresectable disease on first-line therapies by National Comprehensive Cancer Network guidelines.[29]

Oncolytic viral therapies in development
Several other promising oncolytic viruses are currently being evaluated.[40–43] The engineered serotype 5 adenovirus ONCOS-102 has been well tolerated in a phase 1 study and is currently being evaluated in clinical trials in combination with pembrolizumab for unresectable melanoma (NCT03003676).[42,44] Similar to T-VEC, ONCOS-102 has been genetically modified to express GM-CSF to enhance antitumor immunity.[42] Correlative immune studies during the phase 1 trial in refractory solid tumors (although melanoma was not included) found that intralesional treatment with the virus was associated with an increase in systemic proinflammatory cytokines, as well as infiltration of immune cells, particularly $CD8^+$ T cells, into the tumors.[44]

Another promising oncolytic virus is the genetically unaltered coxsackie virus A21 (CVA21, CAVATAK), which preferentially infects tumor cells and causes cell lysis and an enhanced antitumor response.[45] In the phase 2 CALM trial, 57 patients with stage IIIC to IVM1c melanoma received injections of CVA21 on days 1, 3, 5, 8, and 22, and then every 3 weeks for 6 additional injections. Results showed an ORR of 28.1% with a median time to response of 2.8 months, and the study met its primary endpoint of immune-related progression-free survival of 38.6% at 6 months.[45] There were no grade 3 or 4 events, and the most common grade 1 events were fatigue, chills, local injection site reactions, and fever. Ongoing trials are currently investigating CVA21 combinations with pembrolizumab as well as ipilimumab (NCT02565992, NCT02307149). In preliminary data from the initial 23 patients enrolled in the phase 1b MITCI trial combining CVA21 with ipilimumab, there were no dose-limiting toxicities, and the ORR in evaluable patients was 50%.[46]

PVSRIPO is a live-attenuated, recombinant poliovirus type 1 (Sabin) that contains the internal ribosome entry site of human rhinovirus type 2, thus eliminating neurovirulence of the virus.[41] It exhibits tropism for multiple tumor types, including melanoma owing to upregulation of the poliovirus receptor (CD155) on tumor cells, and has shown promise in preclinical models by eliciting an IFN-dominant immune response in the tumor microenvironment, leading to dendritic and T-cell infiltration.[41,47] Intratumoral injection of PVSRIPO has shown promising results in glioblastoma multiforme trials, and a phase 1 trial in refractory melanoma is currently ongoing (NCT03712358).[48] Other ongoing clinical trials include evaluation of a vesicular stomatitis virus modified to contain human IFN-β and TYRP1, an antigen expressed in melanocytes (NCT03865212), and HF10 and RP1, both genetically modified herpes viruses (NCT03259425, NCT03767348).

Melanoma vaccines

Melanoma vaccines aim to overcome tumor immune evasion mechanisms and stimulate an antitumor immune response via delivery of a target antigen or antigens and an adjuvant designed to enhanced immune responses to the vaccine.[49] Vaccines in development have been used as monotherapy or in conjunction with other immunotherapies, such as ICB, to provide synergistic immune activation and improved antitumor efficacy, with the goal of producing a durable, targeted immunologic memory against the tumor to prevent metastasis or recurrence. Melanoma vaccines differ based on the adjuvant provided as well as the type and number of antigens involved, which can be whole cells, including tumor or dendritic cells, tumor lysates, peptides or peptide fragments, RNA, or DNA. Many previously explored vaccine antigens are commonly shared across many melanomas, such as the tumor-associated antigens MAGE-1, MAGE-3, MART-1, glycoprotein 100 (gp100), and tyrosinase.[49] A vaccine incorporating a modified gp100 peptide designed to increase affinity to HLA-A2 has been extensively studied and was evaluated in a phase 3 trial in combination with high-dose IL-2 versus IL-2 alone and showed an improvement in overall clinical response in the vaccine group (16% vs 6%, $P = .03$) as well as a trend toward longer OS (17.8 vs 11.1 months, $P = .06$).[50] However, a subsequent trial combining the vaccine with ipilimumab failed to show that adding the vaccine potentiated the clinical benefits of ipilimumab alone.[51] Another melanoma vaccine is 6-melanoma helper peptide (6-MHP), which combines multiple melanoma peptides derived from cancer-testis antigens and melanocytic differentiation proteins.[52,53] Delivery of the vaccine leads to T-cell and antibody responses in patients with stage III and IV melanoma, which when present were associated with improved survival.[53] Ongoing trials are currently evaluating 6-MHP and other peptide vaccines (NCT03617328, NCT02382549, NCT02515227, NCT02126579).

Recent advances in tumor sequencing technologies have led to significant break-throughs in the development of neoantigen vaccines designed to target personal tumor-specific mutations.[54,55] Two recent landmark studies developed neoantigen vaccines based on algorithms to select personalized immunopeptides predicted to generate immunologic responses from individual melanoma genome mutations.[54,55] Both were able to show that these personalized neoantigen vaccines were able to create robust immune responses to the neoantigens and showed encouraging clinical results in small cohorts of patients. Numerous trials are now ongoing to evaluate these vaccines. Although promising, disadvantages to this approach are the high costs associated, labor-intensive development, and the lag time required to synthesize these vaccines.

Rose bengal

Rose bengal (PV-10) is a 10% solution of rose bengal disodium dye, a fluorescein de-rivative that has been studied extensively and accumulates in lysosomes of tumor cells, leading to autolysis.[56] A phase 1 trial and subsequent phase 2 trial have shown that intralesional injection of PV-10 is well tolerated and can lead to treatment re-sponses in more than 50% of injected lesions as well as a bystander effect with response in noninjected lesions and significant delays in disease progression.[56,57] An international, multicenter phase 2 trial is currently ongoing to evaluate the combi-nation of PV-10 with pembrolizumab (NCT02557321).

Proinflammatory Cytokines

Similar to IL-2 and IFN, which are FDA approved for use in melanoma but rarely used in current clinical practice due to the advent of more effective treatments as well as sig-nificant side effects when delivered systemically, other inflammatory cytokines have been explored for their ability to stimulate an inflammatory tumor microenvironment. IL-12 is a proinflammatory cytokine produced by dendritic cells, macrophages, and neutrophils that has a variety of proinflammatory immunologic functions, including promotion of a T-helper cell 1 response.[58] Early studies evaluating intratumoral injec-tion of IL-12 plasmid DNA in melanoma showed that the local treatment was well toler-ated and leads to reduction of size in a proportion of injected lesions, but did not have an effect on nontreated lesions.[59] Electroporation is being evaluated as a way to improve clinical benefit of IL-12, by permeabilizing cell membranes and increasing transfection of IL-12 DNA plasmids to increase localized IL-12 expression (NCT03132675).[58]

Toll-like receptor agonists

Finally, another encouraging opportunity in injectable therapies for melanoma is the administration of toll-like receptor (TLR) agonists, either as vaccine adjuvants or by direct intratumoral injection. TLR agonists stimulate the innate immune system, leading to production of local cytokines and a proinflammatory response that may lead to more effective antitumor responses. SD-101 and CMP-001 are both TLR9 agonists being investigated in melanoma.[60,61] SD-101, a synthetic CpG oligo-nucleotide, is currently being evaluated in a phase 1b/2 multicenter trial in combi-nation with pembrolizumab for patients with unresectable or metastatic melanoma (NCT02521870). In the first phase of the dose escalation, trial injections were generally well tolerated and led to a 78% ORR in patients naïve to anti-PD-1 ther-apy and a 15% ORR in patients that had prior anti-PD-1 therapy, with responses seen in noninjected, distant lesions.[60] Immune expression profiling showed an increase in tumor infiltrates with CD4[+] and CD8[+] T cells, supporting the conversion of a cold to hot tumor microenvironment. Similarly, CMP-001, a CpG-A oligodeoxynucleotide encapsulated in a viruslike particle, is another TLR9 agonist that showed early promise in an interim analysis of a phase 1b study combining CMP-001 with pembrolizumab in 68 patients with advanced melanoma resistant to anti-PD-1 therapy.[61] Ongoing trials will further evaluate the safety and efficacy of TLR agonists (NCT02521870, NCT03084640, NCT03618641, NCT02680184, NCT02668770, NCT03445533).

SUMMARY

Injectable therapies for melanoma are attractive because of the ease of intralesional delivery to cutaneous, subcutaneous, and nodal metastases, limited systemic toxicity profiles, and importantly, the ability to convert cold, noninflamed tumors into hot, inflamed tumors that may have better responses to systemic therapies.[62] As lack of T-cell infiltration into the tumor microenvironment can be both a barrier to and a predictor of response to ICB, there is significant interest in overcoming this immune evasion mechanism and modulating the tumor microenvironment.[63] Intralesional injection with oncolytic viruses such as T-VEC, immune modulators such as TLR agonists or inflammatory cytokines as well as numerous other substances under investigation can promote an inflammatory response in the tumor microenvironment. Although multiple injectable treatments have been shown to have the ability to cause local antitumor effects, such as direct cytotoxicity, local immune cell infiltration, and clinical responses in injected lesions, the most promising intralesional therapies also lead to a systemic antitumor immune response, causing responses in distant as well as injected lesions, particularly when combined with systemic therapy. Indeed, most ongoing trials evaluating intralesional therapies are in combination with ICB and targeted therapies.

In the current landscape of melanoma treatment, in which better responses to novel treatments are being seen more than ever before, injectable therapies can be considered part of a multifaceted approach to patients with IT melanoma as well as unresectable locally advanced and metastatic melanoma. The only FDA-approved injectable therapy in wide clinical use currently is T-VEC, although there are many others being evaluated in the clinical trial setting. Although injectable therapies as monotherapy have not yet been shown to lead to an improvement in melanoma-specific or overall survival, they can be beneficial in subsets of patients.[26,35,64]

In patients with rapidly progressive disease, the use of locoregional therapies, such as intralesional therapy or regional chemotherapy, must be weighed with the risk of the development of distant metastases, and systemic therapies are often the preferred first-line therapy. However, intralesional therapies may be used in patients with recurrent disease, those who have failed systemic therapy, or those who are not candidates for systemic therapy. Special consideration for injectable therapies may be given to patients who are frail or have multiple comorbidities and may not be able to tolerate systemic therapies and their requisite side effects, as well as in a palliative setting to improve quality of life, or for patients not interested in systemic therapies or morbid surgical resection. Future use of injectable therapies will likely be in conjunction with other systemic therapies or in sequence with surgical therapy to downstage tumors or prevent recurrence. Ongoing trials investigating novel intralesional therapies as well as the synergistic benefits of combination therapies will better guide which patients will benefit most from intralesional therapies in the future.

DISCLOSURE

The authors have no disclosures related to this work. To the best of the authors' knowledge, this review contains no material previously published or written by another person except where due references are made. There was no funding provided for this work.

REFERENCES

1. Read RL, Haydu L, Saw RP, et al. In-transit melanoma metastases: incidence, prognosis, and the role of lymphadenectomy. Ann Surg Oncol 2015;22(2): 475–81.
2. Pawlik TM, Ross MI, Johnson MM, et al. Predictors and natural history of in-transit melanoma after sentinel lymphadenectomy. Ann Surg Oncol 2005;12(8):587–96.
3. Haydu LE, Scolyer RA, Lo S, et al. Conditional survival: an assessment of the prognosis of patients at time points after initial diagnosis and treatment of locoregional melanoma metastasis. J Clin Oncol 2017;35(15):1721–9.
4. Gershenwald JE, Scolyer RA. Melanoma staging: American Joint Committee on Cancer (AJCC) 8th edition and beyond. Ann Surg Oncol 2018;25(8):2105–10.
5. Vilain RE, Menzies AM, Wilmott JS, et al. Dynamic changes in PD-L1 expression and immune infiltrates early during treatment predict response to PD-1 blockade in melanoma. Clin Cancer Res 2017;23(17):5024–33.
6. Topalian SL, Taube JM, Anders RA, et al. Mechanism-driven biomarkers to guide immune checkpoint blockade in cancer therapy. Nat Rev Cancer 2016;16(5): 275–87.
7. Miura JT, Kroon HM, Beasley GM, et al. Long-term oncologic outcomes after isolated limb infusion for locoregionally metastatic melanoma: an international multicenter analysis. Ann Surg Oncol 2019;26(8):2486–94.
8. Wolchok JD, Chiarion-Sileni V, Gonzalez R, et al. Overall survival with combined nivolumab and ipilimumab in advanced melanoma. N Engl J Med 2017;377(14): 1345–56.
9. Robert C, Ribas A, Schachter J, et al. Pembrolizumab versus ipilimumab in advanced melanoma (KEYNOTE-006): post-hoc 5-year results from an open-label, multicentre, randomised, controlled, phase 3 study. Lancet Oncol 2019; 20(9):1239–51.
10. Gogas HJ, Flaherty KT, Dummer R, et al. Adverse events associated with encorafenib plus binimetinib in the COLUMBUS study: incidence, course and management. Eur J Cancer 2019;119:97–106.
11. Byers BA, Temple-Oberle CF, Hurdle V, et al. Treatment of in-transit melanoma with intra-lesional interleukin-2: a systematic review. J Surg Oncol 2014;110(6): 770–5.
12. Krone B, Kolmel KF, Henz BM, et al. Protection against melanoma by vaccination with bacille Calmette-Guerin (BCG) and/or vaccinia: an epidemiology-based hypothesis on the nature of a melanoma risk factor and its immunological control. Eur J Cancer 2005;41(1):104–17.
13. Danielli R, Patuzzo R, Di Giacomo AM, et al. Intralesional administration of L19-IL2/L19-TNF in stage III or stage IVM1a melanoma patients: results of a phase II study. Cancer Immunol Immunother 2015;64(8):999–1009.
14. Sato-Kaneko F, Yao S, Ahmadi A, et al. Combination immunotherapy with TLR agonists and checkpoint inhibitors suppresses head and neck cancer. JCI insight 2017;2(18) [pii:93397].

15. Karakousis CP, Douglass HO Jr, Yeracaris PM, et al. BCG immunotherapy in patients with malignant melanoma. Arch Surg 1976;111(6):716–8.
16. Morton DL, Eilber FR, Holmes EC, et al. BCG immunotherapy of malignant melanoma: summary of a seven-year experience. Ann Surg 1974;180(4):635–43.
17. Tan JK, Ho VC. Pooled analysis of the efficacy of bacille Calmette-Guerin (BCG) immunotherapy in malignant melanoma. J Dermatol Surg Oncol 1993;19(11): 985–90.
18. Robinson JC. Risks of BCG intralesional therapy: an experience with melanoma. J Surg Oncol 1977;9(6):587–93.
19. Sparks FC, Silverstein MJ, Hunt JS, et al. Complications of BCG immunotherapy in patients with cancer. N Engl J Med 1973;289(16):827–30.
20. Agarwala SS, Neuberg D, Park Y, et al. Mature results of a phase III randomized trial of bacillus Calmette-Guerin (BCG) versus observation and BCG plus dacarbazine versus BCG in the adjuvant therapy of American Joint Committee on Cancer stage I-III melanoma (E1673): a trial of the Eastern Oncology Group. Cancer 2004;100(8):1692–8.
21. Ives NJ, Suciu S, Eggermont AMM, et al. Adjuvant interferon-alpha for the treatment of high-risk melanoma: an individual patient data meta-analysis. Eur J Cancer 2017;82:171–83.
22. Ikic D, Spaventi S, Padovan I, et al. Local interferon therapy for melanoma patients. Int J Dermatol 1995;34(12):872–4.
23. Gaffen SL, Liu KD. Overview of interleukin-2 function, production and clinical applications. Cytokine 2004;28(3):109–23.
24. Atkins MB, Lotze MT, Dutcher JP, et al. High-dose recombinant interleukin 2 therapy for patients with metastatic melanoma: analysis of 270 patients treated between 1985 and 1993. J Clin Oncol 1999;17(7):2105–16.
25. Weide B, Derhovanessian E, Pflugfelder A, et al. High response rate after intratumoral treatment with interleukin-2: results from a phase 2 study in 51 patients with metastasized melanoma. Cancer 2010;116(17):4139–46.
26. Boyd KU, Wehrli BM, Temple CL. Intra-lesional interleukin-2 for the treatment of in-transit melanoma. J Surg Oncol 2011;104(7):711–7.
27. Weide B, Eigentler TK, Pflugfelder A, et al. Intralesional treatment of stage III metastatic melanoma patients with L19-IL2 results in sustained clinical and systemic immunologic responses. Cancer Immunol Res 2014;2(7):668–78.
28. Rafei-Shamsabadi D, Lehr S, von Bubnoff D, et al. Successful combination therapy of systemic checkpoint inhibitors and intralesional interleukin-2 in patients with metastatic melanoma with primary therapeutic resistance to checkpoint inhibitors alone. Cancer Immunol Immunother 2019;68(9):1417–28.
29. Coit DG, Thompson JA, Albertini MR, et al. Cutaneous melanoma, version 2.2019, NCCN clinical practice guidelines in oncology. J Natl Compr Canc Netw 2019; 17(4):367–402.
30. Kaufman HL, Kohlhapp FJ, Zloza A. Oncolytic viruses: a new class of immunotherapy drugs. Nat Rev Drug Discov 2015;14(9):642–62.
31. Liu BL, Robinson M, Han ZQ, et al. ICP34.5 deleted herpes simplex virus with enhanced oncolytic, immune stimulating, and anti-tumour properties. Gene Ther 2003;10(4):292–303.
32. Hu JC, Coffin RS, Davis CJ, et al. A phase I study of OncoVEXGM-CSF, a second-generation oncolytic herpes simplex virus expressing granulocyte macrophage colony-stimulating factor. Clin Cancer Res 2006;12(22):6737–47.
33. Senzer NN, Kaufman HL, Amatruda T, et al. Phase II clinical trial of a granulocyte-macrophage colony-stimulating factor-encoding, second-generation oncolytic

herpesvirus in patients with unresectable metastatic melanoma. J Clin Oncol 2009;27(34):5763–71.

34. Andtbacka RH, Kaufman HL, Collichio F, et al. Talimogene laherparepvec improves durable response rate in patients with advanced melanoma. J Clin Oncol 2015;33(25):2780–8.

35. Andtbacka RHI, Collichio F, Harrington KJ, et al. Final analyses of OPTiM: a randomized phase III trial of talimogene laherparepvec versus granulocyte-macrophage colony-stimulating factor in unresectable stage III-IV melanoma. J Immunother Cancer 2019;7(1):145.

36. Ribas A, Dummer R, Puzanov I, et al. Oncolytic virotherapy promotes intratumoral T cell infiltration and improves anti-pd-1 immunotherapy. Cell 2017;170(6): 1109–19.e10.

37. Chesney J, Puzanov I, Collichio F, et al. Randomized, open-label phase II study evaluating the efficacy and safety of talimogene laherparepvec in combination with ipilimumab versus ipilimumab alone in patients with advanced, unresectable melanoma. J Clin Oncol 2018;36(17):1658–67.

38. Sun L, Funchain P, Song JM, et al. Talimogene laherparepvec combined with anti-PD-1 based immunotherapy for unresectable stage III-IV melanoma: a case series. J Immunother Cancer 2018;6(1):36.

39. Long GV, Dummer R, Ribas A, et al. Efficacy analysis of MASTERKEY-265 phase 1b study of talimogene laherparepvec (T-VEC) and pembrolizumab (pembro) for unresectable stage IIIB-IV melanoma. J Clin Oncol 2016;34(15_suppl):9568.

40. Zamarin D, Holmgaard RB, Subudhi SK, et al. Localized oncolytic virotherapy overcomes systemic tumor resistance to immune checkpoint blockade immunotherapy. Sci Transl Med 2014;6(226):226ra232.

41. Brown MC, Holl EK, Boczkowski D, et al. Cancer immunotherapy with recombinant poliovirus induces IFN-dominant activation of dendritic cells and tumor antigen-specific CTLs. Sci Transl Med 2017;9(408) [pii:eaan4220].

42. Kuryk L, Moller AW, Jaderberg M. Combination of immunogenic oncolytic adenovirus ONCOS-102 with anti-PD-1 pembrolizumab exhibits synergistic antitumor effect in humanized A2058 melanoma huNOG mouse model. Oncoimmunology 2019;8(2):e1532763.

43. Shi SW, Li B, Dong Y, et al. In vitro and clinical studies of gene therapy with recombinant human adenovirus-p53 injection for malignant melanoma. Hum Gene Ther Clin Dev 2019;30(1):7–18.

44. Ranki T, Pesonen S, Hemminki A, et al. Phase I study with ONCOS-102 for the treatment of solid tumors–an evaluation of clinical response and exploratory analyses of immune markers. J Immunother Cancer 2016;4:17.

45. Andtbacka RHI, Curti BD, Kaufman H, et al. Final data from CALM: a phase II study of Coxsackievirus A21 (CVA21) oncolytic virus immunotherapy in patients with advanced melanoma. J Clin Oncol 2015;33(15_suppl):9030.

46. Curti B, Richards J, Hallmeyer S, et al. Abstract CT114: The MITCI (phase 1b) study: a novel immunotherapy combination of intralesional coxsackievirus A21 and systemic ipilimumab in advanced melanoma patients with or without previous immune checkpoint therapy treatment. Cancer Res 2017;77(13 Supplement):CT114.

47. Gao J, Zheng Q, Xin N, et al. CD155, an onco-immunologic molecule in human tumors. Cancer Sci 2017;108(10):1934–8.

48. Desjardins A, Sampson JH, Peters KB, et al. Patient survival on the dose escalation phase of the Oncolytic Polio/Rhinovirus Recombinant (PVSRIPO) against

WHO grade IV malignant glioma (MG) clinical trial compared to historical controls. J Clin Oncol 2016;34. s abstract 2016.

49. Ott PA, Fritsch EF, Wu CJ, et al. Vaccines and melanoma. Hematol Oncol Clin North Am 2014;28(3):559–69.

50. Schwartzentruber DJ, Lawson DH, Richards JM, et al. gp100 peptide vaccine and interleukin-2 in patients with advanced melanoma. N Engl J Med 2011; 364(22):2119–27.

51. Hodi FS, O'Day SJ, McDermott DF, et al. Improved survival with ipilimumab in patients with metastatic melanoma. N Engl J Med 2010;363(8):711–23.

52. Hu Y, Kim H, Blackwell CM, et al. Long-term outcomes of helper peptide vaccination for metastatic melanoma. Ann Surg 2015;262(3):456–64 [discussion: 462–4].

53. Reed CM, Cresce ND, Mauldin IS, et al. Vaccination with melanoma helper peptides induces antibody responses associated with improved overall survival. Clin Cancer Res 2015;21(17):3879–87.

54. Ott PA, Hu Z, Keskin DB, et al. An immunogenic personal neoantigen vaccine for patients with melanoma. Nature 2017;547(7662):217–21.

55. Sahin U, Derhovanessian E, Miller M, et al. Personalized RNA mutanome vaccines mobilize poly-specific therapeutic immunity against cancer. Nature 2017; 547(7662):222–6.

56. Thompson JF, Agarwala SS, Smithers BM, et al. Phase 2 study of intralesional PV-10 in refractory metastatic melanoma. Ann Surg Oncol 2015;22(7):2135–42.

57. Thompson JF, Hersey P, Wachter E. Chemoablation of metastatic melanoma using intralesional Rose Bengal. Melanoma Res 2008;18(6):405–11.

58. Canton DA, Shirley S, Wright J, et al. Melanoma treatment with intratumoral electroporation of tavokinogene telseplasmid (pIL-12, tavokinogene telseplasmid). Immunotherapy 2017;9(16):1309–21.

59. Mahvi DM, Henry MB, Albertini MR, et al. Intratumoral injection of IL-12 plasmid DNA–results of a phase I/IB clinical trial. Cancer Gene Ther 2007;14(8):717–23.

60. Ribas A, Medina T, Kummar S, et al. SD-101 in combination with pembrolizumab in advanced melanoma: results of a phase ib, multicenter study. Cancer Discov 2018;8(10):1250–7.

61. Milhem MM, Gonzalez R, Medina T, et al. Intratumoral toll-like receptor 9 (TLR9) agonist, CMP-001, in combination with pembrolizumab can reverse resistance to PD-1 inhibition in a phase Ib trial in subjects with advanced melanoma. Proceedings of the 109th Annual Meeting of the American Association for Cancer Research:Chicago, IL. April 14–18, 2018.

62. Ott PA. Intralesional cancer immunotherapies. Hematol Oncol Clin North Am 2019;33(2):249–60.

63. Fridman WH, Zitvogel L, Sautes-Fridman C, et al. The immune contexture in cancer prognosis and treatment. Nat Rev Clin Oncol 2017;14(12):717–34.

64. Masoud SJ, Hu JB, Beasley GM, et al. Efficacy of talimogene laherparepvec (T-VEC) therapy in patients with in-transit melanoma metastasis decreases with increasing lesion size. Ann Surg Oncol 2019;26(13):4633–41.

Neoadjuvant Therapy for Melanoma

Michael C. Lowe, MD, MA[a],*, Ragini R. Kudchadkar, MD[b]

KEYWORDS

- Melanoma • Immunotherapy • Targeted therapy • Neoadjuvant

KEY POINTS

- Early data from small neoadjuvant clinical trials in melanoma confirm the need to preform larger randomized clinical trials to confirm these results.
- Patients with macroscopically detected resectable stage III disease should receive neoadjuvant therapy on a clinical trial.
- Patients treated with neoadjuvant immunotherapy that experience complete pathologic responses are less likely to relapse in small studies with term short term follow up.

ROLE OF NEOADJUVANT THERAPY IN MELANOMA

Stage III melanoma represents a wide variety of patients, including those with microscopic disease found on sentinel lymph node evaluation as well as those with in-transit or clinically detected lymph nodes at the time of diagnosis. Although both populations are at risk for recurrence, patients with in-transit and clinically detected disease have poorer prognosis. Historically, patients with clinically detected lymph nodes without in-transit metastases have a 5-year recurrence rate of 68% to 89%.[1,2] Patients with stage IIID melanoma (high-risk primary lesion and multiple nodes involved) have prognosis similar to patients with stage IV disease.[3]

For patients with regional disease, conventional management includes excision of the primary and any resectable in-transit disease, if present; therapeutic lymphadenectomy; and adjuvant therapy. Historically adjuvant therapy consisted only of high-dose interferon or ipilimumab.[4,5] These therapies had limited efficacy and high toxicities that limited their widespread use. Recent trials have shown significant improvements in overall survival (OS) and/or recurrence-free survival for Programmed cell death protein-1 (PD-1) inhibitors and BRAF/MEK targeted therapies in the adjuvant setting.[6-8] These improvements, however, over either placebo or ipilimumab

[a] Department of Surgery, Emory University School of Medicine, 1365 Clifton Road, Atlanta, GA 30322, USA; [b] Department of Hematology and Oncology, Winship Cancer Institute, 1365 Clifton Road, Atlanta, GA 30322, USA
* Corresponding author.
E-mail address: mlowe3@emory.edu

Surg Oncol Clin N Am 29 (2020) 445–453
https://doi.org/10.1016/j.soc.2020.03.001
1055-3207/20/© 2020 Elsevier Inc. All rights reserved.

leave a clear unmet need to further improve outcomes. Data in other solid tumors, including breast, bladder, and esophageal, among others, suggest neoadjuvant therapy could have considerable impact on disease response, operability, and survival rates.[9–11] Early studies in melanoma suggest similar results.

This review outlines the current data for both immunotherapy and targeted therapy in the neoadjuvant setting and determines how neoadjuvant therapy should fit into the current paradigm of treatment of patients with resectable clinically detected regional disease.

WHY NEOADJUVANT THERAPY?

Given the advances in both the metastatic and adjuvant settings, neoadjuvant strategies have been the logical next frontier in the treatment of melanoma. Neoadjuvant treatments ideally would improve both recurrence-free survival (RFS) and overall survival (OS) for melanoma patients. Other endpoints, however, potentially will benefit patients even if RFS and OS are not changed. Decreasing surgical morbidity, understanding disease biology/responsiveness to therapy, prognostic data of pathologic response, and perhaps identifying biomarkers to determine future adjuvant therapy are just some of the potential benefits to a neoadjuvant paradigm.

Preclinical evidence has shown that mice treated with neoadjuvant anti–PD-1 antibody prior to resection had a better survival then mice treated after surgery.[12] In addition, tumor resistance can occur via changes to the tumor microenvironment through the course of therapy, thus making earlier treatment a promising paradigm to prevent resistance.

Beyond direct patient benefit, the neoadjuvant paradigm has the potential to promote scientific advancement in the field. If endpoints, such as pathologic complete response (pCR), are established as a predictor of survival, drugs may be tested in the neoadjuvant setting in order to predict outcomes for metastatic patients. This method would be more cost-effective and faster compared with randomized phase III trials. Although a pooled analysis of early neoadjuvant trials in melanoma shows pCR to be a predictor of improved outcomes, data correlating pCR to OS benefit have yet to be established.[13]

NEOADJUVANT IMMUNOTHERAPY

Long-term survival in stage IV melanoma has been seen with anti–PD-1 antibodies as single agents and in combination with cytotoxic T lymphocyte-associated antigen-4 (CTLA-4) antibodies. CheckMate 067 reported a 52% OS of stage IV melanoma patients treated with ipilimumab and nivolumab and 44% OS for patients on nivolumab monotherapy.[14] Similar results have been seen with pembrolizumab monotherapy, with KEYNOTE-001 demonstrating a 5-year OS of 34%.[15] In light of these significant survival improvements in the stage IV setting, use of anti–PD-1 with and without anti–CTLA-4 antibodies have been explored in the neoadjuvant setting (**Table 1**).

Remarkably, even a single dose of pembrolizumab has been shown to elicit a pathologic response in patients with metastatic resectable melanoma. A single-institution trial enrolled 29 patients with resectable stage IIIB, IIIC, and stage IV melanoma, and patients were treated with 1 dose of pembrolizumab and then went to surgical resection. Of 27 patients who were evaluable for pathologic response, 5 had pCR and 3 had a pathologic major response (less than 10% viable tumor). The patients with pCR and pathologic major response remained disease-free at the time of publication.[16] This small study demonstrates the potential prognostic significance of pathologic response.

Nivolumab has also been studied in the neoadjuvant setting as single agent and in combination with ipilimumab. A phase II trial by Amaria and colleagues[17] evaluated neoadjuvant immunotherapy in resectable stage III and stage IV melanoma patients, who were randomized to 2 treatment arms: nivolumab, 3 mg/kg, intravenous, every 2 weeks × 4 cycles prior to resection (n = 11), or ipilimumab, 3 mg/kg, and nivolumab, 1 mg/kg, every 3 weeks for 3 cycles prior to surgery (n = 12). With nivolumab monotherapy, the response evaluation criteria in solid tumors (RECIST) response rate was 25% and pCR was 25%. With combination nivolumab/ipilimumab therapy, the RECIST response was 73% with pCR rate of 45%. The rate of grade 3 or higher adverse events in the nivolumab/ipilimumab combination arm, however, was 73% compared with 8% in the nivolumab only arm.[17]

A phase Ib study by Blank and colleagues[18] evaluated both neoadjuvant and adjuvant immunotherapy in clinical stage III patients only. Patients received either adjuvant ipilimumab (3 mg/kg) plus nivolumab (1 mg/kg) every 3 weeks for 4 cycles after surgery (n = 10) or neoadjuvant ipilimumab plus nivolumab for 2 cycles prior to surgery and another 2 cycles postoperatively (n = 10). On the neoadjuvant arm there were 3 pCRs, 3 patients with major response (less than 10% viable tumor), and 1 patient with partial pathologic response (10%–50% viable tumor). Of the pCR and near-complete response (CR) patients, none had recurred at the time of publication, again suggesting prognostic significance of pCR. On the adjuvant arm, 4 of the 10 patients treated had relapsed at that the time of publication.[18] With small numbers of subjects, it is difficult to make any firm conclusions comparing neoadjuvant to adjuvant therapy from this trial.

Combination therapy clearly has a higher response rate, but with that comes higher rates of toxicity.[14,19] Therefore the OpACIN-neo trial attempted to optimize dosing in order to minimize adverse events. Three neoadjuvant dosing schedules were evaluated: arm A—ipilimumab, 3 mg/kg, plus nivolumab, 1 mg/kg, for 2 cycles; arm B—ipilimumab, 1 mg/kg, plus nivolumab, 3 mg/kg, for 2 cycles; and arm C—ipilimumab, 3 mg/kg, every 2 weeks for 2 cycles followed by nivolumab, 3 mg/kg, every 2 weeks for 2 cycles. Adjuvant therapy was not given on any arm of the study. Thirty patients were enrolled on first 2 arms and 26 patients were enrolled on the third. Serious adverse events (grades 3 and 4) occurred in 40%, 20%, and 50% in the 3 arms, respectively. pCR rates were 47%, 57%, and 65%, respectively. Due to the lower toxicity and comparable pCR rate of arm B (ipilimumab, 1 mg/kg, with nivolumab, 3 mg/kg), this was concluded by the investigators to be the best dosing and schedule.[20]

These 4 trials provide considerable evidence to support the hypothesis that neoadjuvant therapy with proved combinations of immunotherapy will result in high rates of pathologic response. Given the lack of long-term follow-up from any of these studies, correlations between pathologic response and melanoma-specific survival cannot be drawn. Optimizing combinations of immunotherapy and timing/duration of adjuvant therapy will provide further guidance in creating the optimal neoadjuvant therapy schema.

NEOADJUVANT TARGETED THERAPY

Several trials in stage IV melanoma have established that inhibition of the MAP kinase pathway in BRAF-mutated melanoma leads to survival benefit. Although initial studies showed single-agent BRAF inhibition had OS benefit for stage IV patients, a multitude of studies have now established that combination BRAF with MEK inhibitors is superior to single-agent therapy in both progression-free survival and OS. Three different

Table 1
Completed neoadjuvant studies in locally regionally advanced melanoma

Study	No. of Patients	Design	Regimen	Findings
Neoadjuvant immunotherapy				
Huang and colleagues,[16] 2019	30	Phase I, single arm	Pembro, 200 mg, 1 dose followed by surgery after 3 wk; then, q3wk pembro, for 1 y	• 30% complete or near-complete (<10% viable tumor) pathologic response • 1 y RFS of 55%
OpACIN: Blank and colleagues,[18] 2018	20	Phase Ib	Arm A: adjuvant IV ipi, 3 mg/kg q3wk, + IV nivo, 1 mg/kg q3wk for 12 wk Arm B: IV ipi, 3 mg/kg q3wk, + IV nivo, 1 mg/kg q3wk for 6 wk, bracketing surgery	• Neoadjuvant ipi + nivo led to 3 pCR, 4 near-pCR (microscopic metastatic disease) and 1 PR • Grade 3–4 adverse events in 18/20 patients
OpACIN-neo, phase II; 2019[20]	90	Phase II, 3 arms	Arm A: ipi (3 mg/kg) + nivo (1 mg/kg) q3wk for 6 wk before surgery Arm B: ipi (1 mg/kg) + nivo (3 mg/kg) q3wk for 6 wk before surgery Arm C: ipi (3 mg/kg) q3wk for 6 wk followed immediately by nivo, 3 mg/kg q2wk for 4 wk	• Grade 3/4 adverse events: 40% in arm A, 20% in arm B, and 50% in arm C • Complete radiologic response rate: 7% in arm A, 10% in arm B, and 4% in arm C • pCR rate: 47% in arm A, 47% in arm B, and 23% in arm C
Amaria and colleagues,[19] 2018	23	Phase II	Arm A: neoadjuvant nivo, 3 mg/kg IV q2wk × 4 doses, followed by adjuvant nivo, 3 mg/kg IV q2wk × 13 doses Arm B: neoadjuvant nivo, 1 mg/kg + ipi 3 mg/kg q3wk × 3doses, followed by adjuvant nivo, 3 mg/kg IV q2wk × 13 doses	• Arm A: 25% pCR and 25% radiological response rate • Arm B: 45% pCR and 73% radiological response rate • Grade 3 adverse events—8% in arm A vs 73% in arm B

Neoadjuvant targeted therapy

	N	Phase	Treatment	Results
Long and colleagues,[24] 2019	35	Phase II, single arm	Dabrafenib + trametinib × 12 wk before surgery, followed by dabrafenib + trametinib for 40 wk	• 17/35 (49%) had pCR • 2-y RFS 63.3% in patients with pCR
Combi-Neo, Amaria and colleagues,[25] 2018	21	Phase II, double arm	Arm A: 7 patients—surgery + SOC adjuvant therapy Arm B: 14 pts—neoadjuvant dabrafenib + trametinib for 8 wk, adjuvant dabrafenib + trametinib for 44 wk	• Median event-free survival 19.7 mo (arm B) vs 2.9 mo (arm A) • pCR rate of 58% and pathologic partial response rate of 17%

Neoadjuvant oncolytic viral therapy

	N	Phase	Treatment	Results
Andtbacka & Gyorki,[27] 2018	150	Phase II, double arm	Arm A: 6 cycles of neoaduvant T-VEC followed by surgical resection Arm B: upfront surgical resection	• pCR rate of 21% and overall response rate (CR + PR) of 14.7% in arm A • 11 patients in arm A had progressive disease before surgery

Abbreviations: ipi, ipilimumab; IV, intravenous; nivo, nivolumab; pembro, pembrolizumab; PR, partial response; SOC, standard of care.

combination therapies (BRAF inhibitor plus MEK inhibitor) have been approved for the treatment of stage IV BRAF V600–mutated melanoma (vemurafenib plus cobimetinib, dabrafenib plus trametinib, and encorafenib plus binimetinib).[21–23] Dabrafenib and trametinib also have been approved for the treatment of resected stage III melanoma given the improved RFS compared with observation.[7]

Several small studies are available that show activity of these agents in the neoadjuvant setting. In a phase II trial by Long and colleagues,[24] dabrafenib and trametinib was administered to 35 patients with stage IIIB/C BRAF V600E/K–mutated melanoma. Patients were treated for 12 weeks and then underwent therapeutic lymph node dissection followed by 40 weeks of adjuvant targeted therapy. Of the 35 patients, 17 achieved a pCR rate of 49%. At median follow-up of 27 months, recurrence was noted in 20 patients; 2-year RFS was 63.3% in patients with pCR compared with 24.4% in patients who did not achieve pCR. Ten patients (29%) experienced grades 3 to 4 adverse events, most commonly pyrexia.[24]

Amaria and colleagues[25] also evaluated the role of neoadjuvant dabrafenib and trametinib in 21 patients with resectable stage III or oligometastatic stage IV resectable BRAF-mutated melanoma. Patients were randomized in a 1:2 ratio to either upfront surgery followed by standard of care adjuvant dabrafenib/trametinib or neoadjuvant dabrafenib plus trametinib for 8 weeks, followed by surgery, followed by 44 weeks of adjuvant therapy. This trial was stopped early at a predetermined interim analysis because a significant improvement in RFS was noted in the neoadjuvant arm. Of the 12 patients in the neoadjuvant arm, 58% achieved pCR. In addition, as seen in other studies, patients with pCR had a significantly longer distant metastasis–free survival (hazard ratio 0.082; 95% CI 0.001–0.88; $P = .04$).[25]

ONCOLYTIC VIRAL THERAPY

Talimogene laherparepvec (T-VEC) is a genetically modified herpes simplex virus that specifically infects and replicates in human tumor cells. It is approved for the treatment of unresectable stage III and stage IV melanoma and had the highest efficacy in those with limited disease.[26] Given that most patients with resectable melanoma have limited volume of metastatic disease that is potentially injectable, T-VEC was rationally considered for patients with resectable and injectable stage III and stage IV melanoma. A phase II trial randomized 150 patients with resectable melanoma to either surgery or 6 doses of neoadjuvant T-VEC for up to 12 weeks. A pCR rate of 21% was found in patients undergoing neoadjuvant T-VEC and surgery, but 11 patients had progression of disease before planned surgical resection.[27] With a significant portion of patients becoming unresectable and the lower pCR rate compared with other agents in the neoadjuvant space, single-agent T-VEC has more limited utility as a neoadjuvant treatment.

SUMMARY OF EARLY TRIALS

On behalf of the International Neoadjuvant Melanoma Consortium, Menzies and colleagues,[13] completed a pooled analysis of the 6 trials evaluating neoadjuvant immunotherapy or BRAF-targeted therapy. Patients with RECIST measurable and surgically resectable stage III disease who underwent surgery were included in the analysis. A total of 184 patients were pooled; 133 were treated with immunotherapy and 51 were treated with targeted therapy. Overall, pCR was observed in 41% of patients. At median follow-up of 13 months, 44 (24%) experienced a recurrence. Of patients with pCR, 7% experienced a recurrence; all of these recurrences occurred in patient receiving targeted therapy. None of the patients receiving immunotherapy experienced recurrence. One-year RFS was significantly longer in patients experiencing pCR compared with patients without pCR (95% vs 62%, respectively; p<0.001).[13]

Data from the individual trials and this pooled analysis suggest that neoadjuvant therapy provides a high rate of pathologic response and acceptable tolerability. Despite what appears to be an association between pathologic response and RFS, it is not possible to make correlations between pathologic response and long-term outcomes. Ongoing trials, some of which are larger and powered to address the impact of neoadjuvant therapy on survival, may answer broader questions about the more universal application of neoadjuvant therapy in melanoma.

SUMMARY

The neoadjuvant treatment approach to advanced resectable regional disease is the logical next step in the progress that has been made in the treatment of advanced melanoma. The agents available for use in the neoadjuvant setting are safe and effective, and early trial data have confirmed that the overwhelming majority of patients are able to complete surgical resection. A small minority of patients who are unable to complete surgery have developed systemic disease while on neoadjuvant therapy; most clinicians believe that in these unfortunate circumstances an operation would have provided limited, if any, benefit. Ongoing and future clinical trials must balance the toxicities of systemic therapies with the goal of performing a potentially curable operation for all resectable patients.

In addition to the long-term survival impact that is likely to result from neoadjuvant therapies, administering checkpoint blockade and BRAF-targeted therapies before surgical resection offers an incredible amount of histologic and immunologic data. The neoadjuvant approach will enable investigators to test novel drug combinations, including next-generation immune checkpoint blockade targets like TIGIT, Tim-3, Lag-3, and OX40, among others. The ultimate goal is to identify which patients are most likely to benefit from which of the following: neoadjuvant therapy, upfront surgery followed by adjuvant therapy, and definitive systemic therapy. Large studies comparing neoadjuvant with adjuvant therapy already are under way and will definitively determine if all patients with resectable regional melanoma should undergo systemic therapy prior to their definitive operation. Continued work is required to fully characterize the long-term patterns of response to and relapse from neoadjuvant treatment. As neoadjuvant therapy continues to develop, new targets will be identified to increase response rates with less toxicity. Great strides have been made in the treatment of advanced melanoma patients, and this work continues to expand in the neoadjuvant setting. The authors still feel strongly that all patients with resectable regional melanoma should receive neoadjuvant treatment on a clinical trial when feasible. This will build on the tremendous momentum gained to date and ultimately result in an improvement in the prognosis of this historically devastating disease.

DISCLOSURE

The authors have no disclosures.

REFERENCES

1. Manola J, Atkins M, Ibrahim J, et al. Prognostic factors in metastatic melanoma: a pooled analysis of Eastern Cooperative Oncology Group trials. J Clin Oncol 2000; 18(22):3782–93.

2. Romano E, Scordo M, Dusza SW, et al. Site and timing of first relapse in stage III melanoma patients: implications for follow-up guidelines. J Clin Oncol 2010; 28(18):3042–7.

3. Gershenwald JE, Scolyer RA, Hess KR, et al. Melanoma staging: evidence-based changes in the American Joint Committee on Cancer eighth edition cancer staging manual. CA Cancer J Clin 2017;67(6):472–92.

4. Eggermont AM, Chiarion-Sileni V, Grob JJ, et al. Prolonged survival in stage III Melanoma with ipilimumab adjuvant therapy. N Engl J Med 2016;375(19): 1845–55.

5. Kirkwood JM, Ibrahim JG, Sondak VK, et al. High- and low-dose interferon alfa-2b in high-risk melanoma: first analysis of intergroup trial E1690/S9111/C9190. J Clin Oncol 2000;18(12):2444–58.

6. Eggermont AMM, Blank CU, Mandala M, et al. Adjuvant pembrolizumab versus placebo in resected stage III melanoma. N Engl J Med 2018;378(19):1789–801.

7. Long GV, Hauschild A, Santinami M, et al. Adjuvant dabrafenib plus trametinib in stage III BRAF-mutated melanoma. N Engl J Med 2017;377(19):1813–23.

8. Weber J, Mandala M, Del Vecchio M, et al. Adjuvant nivolumab versus ipilimumab in resected stage III or IV melanoma. N Engl J Med 2017;377(19):1824–35.

9. Estevez LG, Gradishar WJ. Evidence-based use of neoadjuvant taxane in operable and inoperable breast cancer. Clin Cancer Res 2004;10(10):3249–61.

10. Grossman HB, Natale RB, Tangen CM, et al. Neoadjuvant chemotherapy plus cystectomy compared with cystectomy alone for locally advanced bladder cancer. N Engl J Med 2003;349(9):859–66.

11. Medical Research Council Oesophageal Cancer Working Group. Surgical resection with or without preoperative chemotherapy in oesophageal cancer: a randomised controlled trial. Lancet 2002;359(9319):1727–33.

12. Liu J, Blake SJ, Yong MC, et al. Improved efficacy of neoadjuvant compared to adjuvant immunotherapy to eradicate metastatic disease. Cancer Discov 2016; 6(12):1382–99.

13. Menzies AM, Rozeman EA, Amaria RN, et al. Pathologic complete response and survival with neoadjuvant therapy in melanoma: a pooled analysis from the International Neoadjuvant Melnaoma Consortium (INMC). J Clin Oncol 2019;37.

14. Larkin J, Chiarion-Sileni V, Gonzalez R, et al. Five-year survival with combined nivolumab and ipilimumab in advanced melanoma. N Engl J Med 2019;381(16): 1535–46.

15. Hamid O, Robert C, Daud A, et al. Five-year survival outcomes for patients with advanced melanoma treated with pembrolizumab in KEYNOTE-001. Ann Oncol 2019;30(4):582–8.

16. Huang AC, Orlowski RJ, Xu X, et al. A single dose of neoadjuvant PD-1 blockade predicts clinical outcomes in resectable melanoma. Nat Med 2019;25(3):454–61.

17. Amaria RN, Menzies AM, Burton EM, et al. Neoadjuvant systemic therapy in melanoma: recommendations of the International Neoadjuvant Melanoma Consortium. Lancet Oncol 2019;20(7):e378–89.

18. Blank CU, Rozeman EA, Fanchi LF, et al. Neoadjuvant versus adjuvant ipilimumab plus nivolumab in macroscopic stage III melanoma. Nat Med 2018;24(11): 1655–61.

19. Amaria RN, Reddy SM, Tawbi HA, et al. Neoadjuvant immune checkpoint blockade in high-risk resectable melanoma. Nat Med 2018;24(11):1649–54.

20. Rozeman EA, Menzies AM, van Akkooi ACJ, et al. Identification of the optimal combination dosing schedule of neoadjuvant ipilimumab plus nivolumab in

macroscopic stage III melanoma (OpACIN-neo): a multicentre, phase 2, randomised, controlled trial. Lancet Oncol 2019;20(7):948–60.

21. Dummer R, Ascierto PA, Gogas HJ, et al. Overall survival in patients with BRAF-mutant melanoma receiving encorafenib plus binimetinib versus vemurafenib or encorafenib (COLUMBUS): a multicentre, open-label, randomised, phase 3 trial. Lancet Oncol 2018;19(10):1315–27.

22. Flaherty KT, Infante JR, Daud A, et al. Combined BRAF and MEK inhibition in melanoma with BRAF V600 mutations. N Engl J Med 2012;367(18):1694–703.

23. Larkin J, Ascierto PA, Dreno B, et al. Combined vemurafenib and cobimetinib in BRAF-mutated melanoma. N Engl J Med 2014;371(20):1867–76.

24. Long GV, Saw RPM, Lo S, et al. Neoadjuvant dabrafenib combined with trametinib for resectable, stage IIIB-C, BRAF(V600) mutation-positive melanoma (NeoCombi): a single-arm, open-label, single-centre, phase 2 trial. Lancet Oncol 2019;20(7):961–71.

25. Amaria RN, Prieto PA, Tetzlaff MT, et al. Neoadjuvant plus adjuvant dabrafenib and trametinib versus standard of care in patients with high-risk, surgically resectable melanoma: a single-centre, open-label, randomised, phase 2 trial. Lancet Oncol 2018;19(2):181–93.

26. Kaufman HL, Bines SD. OPTIM trial: a Phase III trial of an oncolytic herpes virus encoding GM-CSF for unresectable stage III or IV melanoma. Future Oncol 2010; 6(6):941–9.

27. Andtbacka RHI, Reinhard D, DR, Gyorki DE, et al. Interim analysis of a randomized, open-label phase 2 study of talimogene laherparepvec (T-VEC) neoadjuvant treatment (neotx) plus surgery (surgx) vs surgx for resectable stage IIIB-IVM1a melanoma (MEL). J Clin Oncol 2018;36(15):9508.

Adjuvant Therapy for Cutaneous Melanoma

Darryl Schuitevoerder, MBBS, Charles C. Vining, MD, Jennifer Tseng, MD*

KEYWORDS

- Melanoma • Adjuvant therapy • Immunotherapy • Targeted therapy • BRAF • MEK

KEY POINTS

- Immunotherapy (in the form of ipilimumab, nivolumab, and pembrolizumab) in the adjuvant setting for node-positive melanoma has been shown to improve recurrence-free survival.
- Adjuvant radiation therapy can be considered for patients at high risk of regional nodal recurrence; however, its utility in the era of immunotherapy is uncertain.
- Approximately half of patients with metastatic cutaneous melanoma have an activating mutation in the BRAF gene, most commonly located on the V600 residue (90% V600E).
- Adjuvant BRAF/MEK inhibition for patients with activating BRAF mutations has been shown to improve recurrence-free survival as well as reduce the risk of distant metastasis compared with placebo.
- Development of resistance to BRAF inhibitors is common; however, there are emerging data to suggest that BRAF inhibitor resistance may not be permanent, and there may be value to rechallenging select patients with BRAF/MEK inhibition.

INTRODUCTION

Per the National Cancer Institute Web site, adjuvant therapy is defined as any chemotherapy, radiation, targeted, hormone, or biologic therapy given after the primary treatment in order to decrease the risk of disease recurrence.[1] In the setting of residual disease burden or recurrent disease, additional therapy is not considered adjuvant, and discussion of therapy in these situations will not be covered in this review. The current National Comprehensive Cancer Network guidelines recommend consideration of adjuvant therapy for patients with stage III melanoma.[2] However, the benefit of adjuvant therapy needs to be compared with the potential adverse events (AEs) as well as the baseline probability of locoregional disease recurrence and development of metastatic disease. The decision for or against treatment needs to be individually tailored.

Department of Surgery, University of Chicago, 5841 South Maryland Avenue # MC5094, Chicago, IL 60637, USA
* Corresponding author.
E-mail address: jtseng@surgery.bsd.uchicago.edu

Surg Oncol Clin N Am 29 (2020) 455–465
https://doi.org/10.1016/j.soc.2020.02.009
surgonc.theclinics.com

The single most important prognostic factor for patients with cutaneous melanoma remains their sentinel node status.[3] However, the extent of nodal disease, thickness of the primary tumor, as well as whether there is ulceration present have significant prognostic value and need to be taken into consideration.[4,5] This combination of factors determines the current staging system described by The American Joint Committee on Cancer (AJCC). In the AJCC Eighth Edition, the 5-year melanoma-specific survival (MSS) of patients with stage II disease is 90% compared with 77% for stage III disease.[4] However, within these stage groupings there is wide variation with 5-year MSS of stage IIC (ulcerated primary >4 mm thick) being 82%, which is comparable to that of stage IIIC (5-year MSS 83%) and worse than stage IIIA disease (5-year MSS 93%). Currently, clinical trials are underway to determine the efficacy of checkpoint immunotherapy in these high-risk stage II patients.[6,7] Furthermore, in the era of the second Multicenter Selective Lymphadenectomy Trial and the DeCOG trial, which demonstrated that completion lymph node dissection (CLND) for sentinel lymph node–positive disease did not improve MSS, observation of nodal basins is being performed more routinely in lieu of CLND.[8,9] Because MSS for patients with stage III disease varies depending on the extent of nodal involvement, without CLND it may not be possible to as precisely risk-stratify stage III patients. Furthermore, existing clinical trials that support the use of adjuvant therapy in advanced melanoma primarily included stage III patients with completely resected disease.

The current options for adjuvant therapy for melanoma have changed drastically since the development of modern immunotherapy and targeted therapies. Adjuvant therapy can be thought of as falling under 4 broad categories: immunotherapy, targeted therapy, radiation therapy (RT), and chemotherapy.

ADJUVANT IMMUNOTHERAPY IN ADVANCED MELANOMA
Interferon-Alpha

Historically, adjuvant therapy options for melanoma were limited. Interferon-alpha (INF-α) was the first immunotherapeutic agent approved as adjuvant therapy for high-risk melanoma by the Food and Drug Administration (FDA) in 1995.[10] INF-α was shown to have modest benefit, while harboring unfavorable side-effect profiles.[10–18] Grade 3 and 4 toxicities were reported in up to two-thirds[19,20] of patients, and a 2017 meta-analysis including 15 trials showed an improvement in 5-year overall survival (OS) of 3%, with this benefit seemingly limited to patients with ulcerated primary lesions.[21] INF-α has fallen out of favor with the introduction of other immunotherapy agents.

Ipilimumab

Ipilimumab, a monoclonal antibody targeting CTLA-4, has been FDA approved for adjuvant therapy in stage III melanoma since October 2015. The initial study that demonstrated the efficacy of adjuvant ipilimumab was EORTC 18071, a phase 3 clinical trial comparing high-dose ipilimumab, 10 mg/kg, versus placebo every 3 weeks for 4 doses and then every 3 months for up to 3 years.[22,23] The trial showed significant improvements in 5-year recurrence-free survival (RFS; 40.8 vs 30.3%), OS (65.4% vs 54.4%), and distant metastasis–free survival (48.3 vs 38.9%).[23] Immune-related grade 3 or 4 AEs occurred in 41.6% of the patients in the ipilimumab group with 5 patients dying secondary to immune-related AEs.[22,23]

Until recently there were no data directly comparing the efficacy of INF-α to ipilimumab or other immunotherapy. The results of the Intergroup E1609, a phase 3 randomized study comparing high- and low-dose ipilimumab to INF-α, were recently released in abstract form.[24] The results showed a statistically significant improvement in OS with low-dose ipilimumab (3 mg/kg) compared with high-dose IFN (hazard ratio [HR] 0.78, $P = .044$) and a trend toward improved RFS (HR 0.85, 99.4% confidence interval [CI; 0.66, 1.09], $P = .065$). There was no significant difference in either OS or RFS for patients who received high-dose ipilimumab (10 mg/kg) compared with high-dose INF-α. Grade 3 or 4 AEs were noted in 37% of patients treated with 3 mg/kg ipilimumab compared with 58% with 10 mg/kg ipilimumab and 79% with high-dose INF-α with AEs leading to discontinuation of treatment in 35%, 54%, and 20% of patients, respectively.[24]

Nivolumab

Nivolumab, a monoclonal antibody targeting the programmed cell death protein 1 (PD-1), was first approved by the FDA for use as adjuvant therapy for resected stage III and stage IV patients in December 2017.[25] This approval was a result of published data from the CheckMate 238 Trial, a randomized, double-blind, phase 3 trial of patients with completely resected stage IIIB, IIIC, or IV melanoma. Patients were randomized to receive nivolumab (3 mg/kg) every 2 weeks or ipilimumab (10 mg/kg) every 3 weeks for 4 doses and then every 12 weeks for up to 1 year. The 1-year RFS was 70.5% versus 60.8% (HR 0.65, $P<.001$) favoring the nivolumab group. Furthermore, there was less grade 3 or 4 toxicity noted in the nivolumab group (14.4% vs 45.9%) and a lower rate of treatment discontinuation because of AEs (9.7% vs 42.6%).[26] Updated results from this trial continued to show improved RFS with nivolumab over ipilimumab, with minimum follow-up extended to 24 months.[27]

Pembrolizumab

More recently, another checkpoint inhibitor, pembrolizumab, a monoclonal antibody targeting PD-1, was approved by the FDA for adjuvant therapy in patients with completely resected node-positive disease.[28] This approval was based on data from KEYNOTE-054, which randomized patients with completely resected stage III disease to receive either pembrolizumab or placebo.[29] Patients received 200 mg of pembrolizumab or placebo intravenously every 3 weeks for 1 year, until disease recurrence or therapy was discontinued because of AEs. At median follow-up of 15 months, the pembrolizumab group had significantly improved RFS compared with the placebo group (75% vs 61%, $P<.001$). Grade 3 or higher AEs were reported in 15% of patients treated with pembrolizumab.[29]

SWOG S1404 is an active phase 3 randomized controlled trial comparing the efficacy of pembrolizumab with either ipilimumab or high-dose INF-α. Patients with stage IIIA (N2), IIIB, IIIC, or IV (M1a, b, and c) disease are eligible for enrollment. Primary outcomes are OS and RFS.[30] This trial will provide a head-to-head comparison of pembrolizumab against 2 other immunotherapy options that have been shown to be active in advanced melanoma.[22–24]

Safety of Checkpoint Immunotherapy

Randomized trials examining the efficacy of checkpoint inhibition with adjuvant nivolumab or pembrolizumab have demonstrated less toxicity compared with ipilimumab.[22,24,26,29] The most common AEs are fatigue, skin reactions (rash, pruritis), diarrhea, nausea, arthralgias, and endocrinopathies. The incidence of grade 3 or 4 treatment-related AEs occurred in approximately 46% of the patients treated with high-dose ipilimumab, compared with 14.4% for nivolumab, and 14.7% for pembrolizumab.[23,26,29] The incidence of grade 5 toxicity was also lower in pembrolizumab and nivolumab compared with ipilimumab (0.2%, 0%, and 0.4%–1.1%, respectively).

The most common grade 3 or higher immune-related AEs were gastrointestinal (colitis), endocrine (diabetes mellitus, hypophysitis), and pulmonary/thoracic (pneumonitis, interstitial lung disease).[23,26,29]

ADJUVANT-TARGETED THERAPY IN ADVANCED MELANOMA
BRAF Pathway and Cutaneous Melanoma Implications

Melanoma is a heterogenous malignancy that can be broadly divided into 4 categories based on the mutational profile: BRAF mutant, NRAS mutant, NF1 mutant, and wild type.[31] BRAF is a serine-threonine protein kinase that is responsible for signal transduction within the cell and for normal cell growth, proliferation, differentiation, and survival.[32] Activation of BRAF is via the upstream RAS GTPase protein, which then subsequently activates the downstream ERK pathway.[32–34] Approximately half of patients with metastatic cutaneous melanoma have an activating mutation in the BRAF gene, leading to a constitutively active mitogen-activated protein kinase intracellular pathway.[33,35,36] Most activating mutations are located on the V600 residue, most commonly V600E (90%), but sometimes V600K or others.[36,37] Melanomas that harbor the V600E mutation are active independent of upstream signaling molecules, ultimately leading to cell survival, proliferation, tumor angiogenesis, and metastasis.[33,34] Because of this common mutation, BRAF inhibition (BRAFi) has become a target for intervention.

BRAF-Targeted Therapy

Multiple trials have investigated the efficacy of adjuvant BRAFi in patients with melanoma. In particular, 2 prospective, double-blind, randomized controlled trials have looked at the benefit of adjuvant BRAFi in patients with resected melanoma.[38,39] The BRIM8 trial included patients with AJCC, Seventh Edition stage IIC–III (IIIA with at least 1 lymph node metastasis >1 mm in diameter or stage IIIB/C without in-transit disease) resected melanoma with a BRAF V600 mutation. The use of single-agent vemurafenib versus placebo improved 2-year disease-free survival (62% vs 53%; HR 0.65 [0.50–0.96], P = .0013) and 2-year distant metastasis-free survival (72% vs 65%; HR 0.70 [0.52–0.96], P = .027), but the effect on 2-year OS was not statistically significant (90% vs 86%; HR 0.76 [0.49–1.18], P = .2165).[38] The COMBI-AD trial included patients with resected AJCC, Seventh Edition stage III (IIIA with at least 1 lymph node metastasis >1 mm in diameter or stage IIIB/C) disease with BRAF V600E/K mutation. Patients were randomized to BRAF/MEK inhibitor combination dabrafenib/trametinib versus placebo and demonstrated improved 3-year RFS (58% vs 39%; HR 0.47 [0.40–0.65], P<.001), and reduced risk of distant metastasis (25% vs 35%; HR 0.51 [0.40–0.65], P<.001). The 3-year OS was higher in the dabrafenib/trametinib group (85% vs 77%; HR 0.57 [0.42–0.79], P = .0006) but did not meet the pre-specified interim boundary. A subgroup analysis showed significantly better RFS in patients treated with dabrafenib/trametinib versus placebo in those with BRAF V600E.[39] Based on the COMBI-AD trial, the FDA-approved dabrafenib/trametinib combination therapy for all patients with resected stage III or recurrent disease who have the BRAF V600 activating mutation. Adjuvant combination BRAF/MEK inhibitor therapy should be considered for all patients with stage III melanoma with a BRAF activating mutation.

Presently, adjuvant BRAF inhibitor treatment is not recommended for patients with stage I/II disease. For patients with high-risk stage II disease, clinical trials can be considered and are currently under investigation regarding the role of checkpoint immunotherapy in this setting.[6,7] Enrollment in clinical trials for those with high risk of recurrence after lymphadenectomy or borderline resectable lymphadenopathy should be considered. There are insufficient data regarding BRAF-targeted therapy in the neoadjuvant setting for early-stage melanoma. Neoadjuvant BRAF-targeted therapy for patients with resectable stage III/IV disease has shown promising results and is currently under investigation.[40–45]

Safety of BRAF/MEK Inhibitors

Both BRAFi monotherapy and BRAF/MEK combination therapy demonstrate similar risk profiles with grade 3 to 5 toxicities. In particular, both BRAF monotherapy and BRAF/MEK inhibitor combination therapy are associated with high rates of flulike symptoms, including pyrexia, chills, fatigue, headaches, arthralgias, myalgias, and gastrointestinal symptoms (eg, diarrhea, nausea, vomiting). BRAF/MEK inhibitor combination is associated with higher rates of pyrexia and diarrhea, whereas BRAF monotherapy is associated with increased rates of musculoskeletal complaints. Alopecia, rash, and other skin toxicities are common in both BRAF and BRAF/MEK therapies with occurrence ranging from 6% to 73%.[39,46–49] Notably, BRAFi monotherapy is associated with increased risk of hyperproliferative skin toxicities, including hyperkeratosis, palmoplantar disorders, keratoacanthoma, and cutaneous squamous cell carcinomas compared with BRAF/MEK combination therapy. Specifically, in the BRIM-8 trial, adjuvant vemurafenib was associated with an increase in hyperproliferative cutaneous AE compared with placebo (16% vs 2%).[38] This increase in hyperproliferative cutaneous AEs was not seen in the dabrafenib/trametinib combination therapy as it was with vemurafenib monotherapy.[9] Therefore, the FDA has not approved vemurafenib monotherapy because of the improved efficacy and safety of BRAF/MEK inhibitor combination.

Grade V toxicities are rare in both BRAFi monotherapy and BRAF/MEK combination and include cardiovascular, cerebrovascular, infection, and multiorgan failure events. There are certain rare patients who experience toxicity attributed to MEK inhibition, including deep venous thrombosis, retinal problems, and immunosuppression. In these situations, combination therapy should be discontinued. Other reported AEs include QT prolongation, decreased ejection fraction, and the development of new primary malignancies.[46–50]

Most AEs related to BRAF-targeted therapy manifest within the first few months of therapy, although they can continue throughout the course of treatment. Although time to onset of AEs varies, there is some evidence that development of grade 3 or 4 toxicity was longer in the BRAF/MEK combination therapy group. Most AEs related to treatment toxicity resolved within 3 months of discontinuing therapy.[51–54]

Resistance to BRAF Inhibitors

BRAFi resistance has been shown to be related to the reactivation of the MAP kinase signaling pathway via additional mutations.[55–58] Other mechanisms of resistance involve upregulation of the PI3K-ATK-mTOR signaling, increased expression of growth factor receptors on the cell membrane, amplification or activation of target kinases, and other unknown mechanisms.[58–60] Once BRAF-mutant melanomas become resistant to BRAF inhibitors, their ability to metastasize is increased, and they are more likely to be aggressive with higher rates of progression.[55] There are emerging data to suggest that BRAFi resistance may not be permanent. Phase 1/2 trials evaluating the response to dual BRAF/MEK inhibition after initial progression on BRAFi alone or combination BRAF/MEK inhibition show a relative risk of 13% to 32%, suggesting that BRAF-targeted resistance may be reversible.[61–63] The best patient selection for re-treatment is under investigation; additional questions remain about timing, sequence, and optimal drug selection when treating patients who have progressed after first-line therapy.

Radiation Therapy

Adjuvant RT after wide local excision (WLE) of primary tumors is generally unnecessary because local recurrence after excision with adequate margin has low recurrence rates (1%–9% depending on site of primary).[64] Desmoplastic neurotropic melanomas (DNM) have been associated with higher rates of local recurrence after WLE, and data suggest adjuvant radiation in this setting can be helpful. A retrospective review looking at 128 patients with DNM (27 receiving RT) showed similar rates of local recurrence (6% vs 7% with RT) despite those patients having less favorable clinicopathologic features.[65] Strom and colleagues[66] reported on 277 patients with DNM, of which 113 (40.8%) received adjuvant RT. On multivariable analysis, RT was associated with better local control (HR 0.15, CI 0.06–0.39, $P<.01$) after a mean follow-up of 43 months. Subgroup analysis of 35 patients with positive margin showed a local recurrence rate of 14% in patients who received RT compared with 54% in patients not receiving RT ($P = .004$). For patients with negative resection margin, RT was no longer significant in reducing the local recurrence rate ($P = .09$). However, for those patients with negative margins and high-risk features, thickness greater than 4 mm, head and neck location, on univariate analysis RT was found to significantly reduce the rate of local recurrence ($P<.05$). These data are further supported by a retrospective review of 130 patients with DNM treated at MD Anderson Cancer Center. The authors found that the rate of local recurrence in patients receiving adjuvant RT was significantly lower than for patients with surgery alone (7% vs 24%). On multivariable analysis, RT remained a significant determinant of disease recurrence ($P = .009$).[67] Although these data are promising, they are limited by their single-institution experience and retrospective nature, and randomized trials are needed to definitely determine which patients with DNM benefit from adjuvant RT. Study NCT00975520 is currently accruing and should aid in further defining the role of adjuvant therapy in DNM.[68]

There has been 1 prospective phase 3 randomized controlled trial looking at the utility of adjuvant nodal RT after lymphadenectomy. The ANZMTG 01.02/TROG 02.01 trial randomized 123 patients to adjuvant RT and 127 to observation. After median follow-up of 73 months, nodal relapse occurred in 23 (21%) of the adjuvant RT group compared with 39 (36%) in the observation group (HR 0·52, CI [0.31–0.88], $P = .023$). There was no difference in OS or RFS between the 2 groups. Grade 3 to 4 toxic adverse events were experienced in 22% of the RT group.[69] This outcome is supported by similar results in a large retrospective analysis by Agrawal and colleagues.[70] They examined 615 patients who had undergone lymphadenectomy for metastatic melanoma with 509 (83%) receiving adjuvant RT. At median follow-up of 60 months, patients who received adjuvant RT were less likely to develop a regional nodal recurrence compared with patients who were observed after resection (10.2% vs 40.6%). On multivariable analysis, RT was significantly associated with lower risk of regional recurrence. At 5-year follow-up, the rate of lymphedema was 19%.[70]

Although these data suggest a potential benefit to adjuvant RT in well-selected patients, most data are from before the era of immunotherapy. Treatment with immunotherapy after lymphadenectomy in patients who otherwise would have been considered for adjuvant nodal radiation may potentially limit its benefit because the expected rate of nodal recurrence is much lower. Thus, it would seem reasonable to first treat with immunotherapy when appropriate and reserve RT for salvage rather than adjuvant therapy.

REFERENCES

1. NCI dictionary of cancer terms. Available at: https://www.cancer.gov/publications/dictionaries/cancer-terms/def/adjuvant-therapy. Accessed September 29, 2019.
2. National Comprehensive Cancer Network. Cutaneous melanoma (version 2.2019). Available at: http://www.nccn.org/professionals/physician_gls/pdf/cutaneous_melano ma.pdf. Accessed September 10, 2019.
3. Morton DL, Thompson JF, Cochran AJ, et al. Final trial report of sentinel-node biopsy versus nodal observation in melanoma. N Engl J Med 2014;370(7):599–609.
4. Gershenwald JE, Scolyer RA, Hess KR, et al. Melanoma staging: evidence-based changes in the American Joint Committee on Cancer eighth edition cancer staging manual. CA Cancer J Clin 2017;67(6):472–9.
5. Gershenwald J, Scolyer R, Hess K, et al. AJCC cancer staging manual. Switzerland: Springer; 2017. p. 563–89.
6. Safety and efficacy of pembrolizumab compared to placebo in resected high-risk stage II melanoma (MK-3475-716/KEYNOTE-716). Available at: ClinicalTrials.gov https://clinicaltrials.gov/ct2/show/NCT03553836. Accessed September 15, 2019.
7. Nivolumab in treating patients with stage IIB-IIC melanoma that can be removed by surgery. Available at: ClinicalTrials.gov https://clinicaltrials.gov/ct2/show/record/NCT03405155. Accessed September 15, 2019.
8. Faries MB, Thompson JF, Cochran AJ, et al. Completion dissection or observation for sentinel-node metastasis in melanoma. N Engl J Med 2017;376(23):2211–22.
9. Leiter U, Stadler R, Mauch C, et al. Complete lymph node dissection versus no dissection in patients with sentinel lymph node biopsy positive melanoma (DeCOG-SLT): a multicentre, randomised, phase 3 trial. Lancet Oncol 2016;17(6):757–67.
10. Kirkwood JM, Manola J, Ibrahim J, et al. A pooled analysis of Eastern Cooperative Oncology Group and intergroup trials of adjuvant high-dose interferon for melanoma. Clin Cancer Res 2004;10(5):1670–7.
11. Garbe C, Radny P, Linse R, et al. Adjuvant low-dose interferon {alpha}2a with or without dacarbazine compared with surgery alone: a prospective-randomized phase III DeCOG trial in melanoma patients with regional lymph node metastasis. Ann Oncol 2008;19(6):1195–2001.
12. Eggermont AM, Suciu S, Santinami M, et al. Adjuvant therapy with pegylated interferon alfa-2b versus observation alone in resected stage III melanoma: final results of EORTC 18991, a randomised phase III trial. Lancet 2008;372(9633):117–26.
13. Cascinelli N, Belli F, MacKie RM, et al. Effect of long-term adjuvant therapy with interferon alpha-2a in patients with regional node metastases from cutaneous melanoma: a randomised trial. Lancet 2001;358(9285):866–9.
14. Hancock BW, Wheatley K, Harris S, et al. Adjuvant interferon in high-risk melanoma: the AIM HIGH Study–United Kingdom Coordinating Committee on Cancer Research randomized study of adjuvant low-dose extended-duration interferon Alfa-2a in high-risk resected malignant melanoma. J Clin Oncol 2004;22(1):53–61.
15. Eggermont AM, Suciu S, Rutkowski P, et al. Long term follow up of the EORTC 18952 trial of adjuvant therapy in resected stage IIB-III cutaneous melanoma patients comparing intermediate doses of interferon-alpha-2b (IFN) with observation: ulceration of primary is key determinant for IFN-sensitivity. Eur J Cancer 2016;55:111–21.

16. McMasters KM, Egger ME, Edwards MJ, et al. Final results of the Sunbelt Melanoma Trial: a multi-institutional prospective randomized phase III study evaluating the role of adjuvant high-dose interferon alfa-2b and completion lymph node dissection for patients staged by sentinel lymph node biopsy. J Clin Oncol 2016;34(10):1079–86.

17. Agarwala SS, Lee SJ, Yip W, et al. Phase III randomized study of 4 weeks of high-dose interferon-alpha-2b in stage T2bNO, T3a-bNO, T4a-bNO, and T1-4N1a-2a (microscopic) melanoma: a trial of the Eastern Cooperative Oncology Group-American College of Radiology Imaging Network Cancer Research Group (E1697). J Clin Oncol 2017;35(8):885–92.

18. Hansson J, Aamdal S, Bastholt L, et al. Two different durations of adjuvant therapy with intermediate-dose interferon alfa-2b in patients with high-risk melanoma (Nordic IFN trial): a randomised phase 3 trial. Lancet Oncol 2011;12(2):144–52.

19. Oliver DE, Sondak VK, Strom T, et al. Interferon is associated with improved survival for node-positive cutaneous melanoma: a single-institution experience. Melanoma Manag 2018;5(1):MMT02.

20. Mocellin S, Pasquali S, Rossi CR, et al. Interferon alpha adjuvant therapy in patients with high-risk melanoma: a systematic review and meta-analysis. J Natl Cancer Inst 2010;102(7):493–501.

21. Ives NJ, Suciu S, Eggermont AMM, et al. Adjuvant interferon-alpha for the treatment of high-risk melanoma: an individual patient data meta-analysis. Eur J Cancer 2017;82:171–83.

22. Eggermont AM, Chiarion-Sileni V, Grob JJ, et al. Adjuvant ipilimumab versus placebo after complete resection of high-risk stage III melanoma (EORTC 18071): a randomised, double-blind, phase 3 trial. Lancet Oncol 2015;16(5):522–30.

23. Eggermont AM, Chiarion-Sileni V, Grob JJ, et al. Prolonged survival in stage III melanoma with ipilimumab adjuvant therapy. N Engl J Med 2016;375(19): 1845–55.

24. Tarhini AA, Lee SJ, Hodi FS, et al. United States intergroup E1609: a phase III randomized study of adjuvant ipilimumab (3 or 10 mg/kg) versus high-dose interferon-α2b for resected high-risk melanoma. J Clin Oncol 2019;37(15_suppl): 9504.

25. FDA grants regular approval to nivolumab for adjuvant treatment of melanoma. Available at: https://www.fda.gov/drugs/resources-information-approved-drugs/fda-grants-regular-approval-nivolumab-adjuvant-treatment-melanoma. Accessed September 29, 2019.

26. Weber J, Mandala M, Del Vecchio M, et al. Adjuvant nivolumab versus ipilimumab in resected stage III or IV melanoma. N Engl J Med 2017;377(19):1824–35.

27. Weber JS, Mandalà M, Vecchio MD, et al. Adjuvant therapy with nivolumab (NIVO) versus ipilimumab (IPI) after complete resection of stage III/IV melanoma: updated results from a phase III trial (CheckMate 238). J Clin Oncol 2018; 36(15_suppl):9502.

28. FDA approves pembrolizumab for adjuvant treatment of melanoma. Available at: https://www.fda.gov/drugs/drug-approvals-and-databases/fda-approves-pembrolizumab-adjuvant-treatment-melanoma. Accessed October 2, 2019.

29. Eggermont AMM, Blank CU, Mandala M, et al. Adjuvant pembrolizumab versus placebo in resected stage iii melanoma. N Engl J Med 2018;378(19):1789–801.

30. High-dose recombinant interferon alfa-2B, ipilimumab, or pembrolizumab in treating patients with stage III-IV high risk melanoma that has been removed by surgery. Available at: ClinicalTrials.gov https://clinicaltrials.gov/ct2/show/NCT 02506153?term=S1404&rank=1. Accessed September 29, 2019.

31. Cancer Genome Atlas Network. Genomic Classification of Cutaneous Melanoma. Cell 2015;161(7):1681–96. https://doi.org/10.1016/j.cell.2015.05.044.
32. Fisher R, Larkin J. Vemurafenib: a new treatment for BRAF-V600 mutated advanced melanoma. Cancer Manag Res 2012;4:243–52. https://doi.org/10.2147/CMAR.S25284.
33. Dhillon AS, Hagan S, Rath O, et al. MAP kinase signalling pathways in cancer. Oncogene 2007;26(22):3279–90.
34. Muthusamy VPT. Melanoma cell signalling: looking beyond RAS-RAF-MEK. In: Porta CAML, editor. Skin cancers-risk factors, prevention and therapy. Rijeka (Croatia): InTech; 2011. p. 87–98.
35. Davies H, Bignell GR, Cox C, et al. Mutations of the BRAF gene in human cancer. Nature 2002;417(6892):949–54.
36. Long GV, Menzies AM, Nagrial AM, et al. Prognostic and clinicopathologic associations of oncogenic BRAF in metastatic melanoma. J Clin Oncol 2011;29(10): 1239–46.
37. Ekedahl H, Cirenajwis H, Harbst K, et al. The clinical significance of BRAF and NRAS mutations in a clinic-based metastatic melanoma cohort. Br J Dermatol 2013;169(5):1049–55.
38. Maio M, Lewis K, Demidov L, et al. Adjuvant vemurafenib in resected, BRAF(V600) mutation-positive melanoma (BRIM8): a randomised, double-blind, placebo-controlled, multicentre, phase 3 trial. Lancet Oncol 2018;19(4):510–20.
39. Long GV, Hauschild A, Santinami M, et al. Adjuvant dabrafenib plus trametinib in stage III BRAF-mutated melanoma. N Engl J Med 2017;377(19):1813–23.
40. Amaria RN, Prieto PA, Tetzlaff MT, et al. Neoadjuvant plus adjuvant dabrafenib and trametinib versus standard of care in patients with high-risk, surgically resectable melanoma: a single-centre, open-label, randomised, phase 2 trial. Lancet Oncol 2018;19(2):181–93.
41. Blank CU, Rozeman EA, Fanchi LF, et al. Neoadjuvant versus adjuvant ipilimumab plus nivolumab in macroscopic stage III melanoma. Nat Med 2018;24(11): 1655–61.
42. Amaria RN, Reddy SM, Tawbi HA, et al. Neoadjuvant immune checkpoint blockade in high-risk resectable melanoma. Nat Med 2018;24(11):1649–54.
43. Tarhini AA, Edington H, Butterfield LH, et al. Immune monitoring of the circulation and the tumor microenvironment in patients with regionally advanced melanoma receiving neoadjuvant ipilimumab. PLoS One 2014;9(2):e87705.
44. Retseck J, VanderWeele R, Lin HM, et al. Phenotypic and functional testing of circulating regulatory T cells in advanced melanoma patients treated with neoadjuvant ipilimumab. J Immunother Cancer 2016;4:38.
45. Tarhini AA, Zahoor H, Lin Y, et al. Baseline circulating IL-17 predicts toxicity while TGF-beta1 and IL-10 are prognostic of relapse in ipilimumab neoadjuvant therapy of melanoma. J Immunother Cancer 2015;3:39.
46. Robert C, Karaszewska B, Schachter J, et al. Improved overall survival in melanoma with combined dabrafenib and trametinib. N Engl J Med 2015;372(1):30–9.
47. Dummer R, Ascierto PA, Gogas HJ, et al. Overall survival in patients with BRAF-mutant melanoma receiving encorafenib plus binimetinib versus vemurafenib or encorafenib (COLUMBUS): a multicentre, open-label, randomised, phase 3 trial. Lancet Oncol 2018;19(10):1315–27.
48. Ascierto PA, McArthur GA, Dreno B, et al. Cobimetinib combined with vemurafenib in advanced BRAF(V600)-mutant melanoma (coBRIM): updated efficacy results from a randomised, double-blind, phase 3 trial. Lancet Oncol 2016;17(9): 1248–60.

49. Long GV, Flaherty KT, Stroyakovskiy D, et al. Dabrafenib plus trametinib versus dabrafenib monotherapy in patients with metastatic BRAF V600E/K-mutant melanoma: long-term survival and safety analysis of a phase 3 study. Ann Oncol 2017; 28(7):1631–9.

50. Blank CU, Larkin J, Arance AM, et al. Open-label, multicentre safety study of vemurafenib in 3219 patients with BRAF(V600) mutation-positive metastatic melanoma: 2-year follow-up data and long-term responders' analysis. Eur J Cancer 2017;79:176–84.

51. Larkin J, Del Vecchio M, Ascierto PA, et al. Vemurafenib in patients with BRAF(V600) mutated metastatic melanoma: an open-label, multicentre, safety study. Lancet Oncol 2014;15(4):436–44.

52. Dummer R, Ascierto PA, Gogas HJ, et al. Encorafenib plus binimetinib versus vemurafenib or encorafenib in patients with BRAF-mutant melanoma (COLUMBUS): a multicentre, open-label, randomised phase 3 trial. Lancet Oncol 2018;19(5): 603–15.

53. Long GV, Eroglu Z, Infante J, et al. Long-term outcomes in patients with BRAF V600-mutant metastatic melanoma who received dabrafenib combined with trametinib. J Clin Oncol 2018;36(7):667–73.

54. Dreno B, Ribas A, Larkin J, et al. Incidence, course, and management of toxicities associated with cobimetinib in combination with vemurafenib in the coBRIM study. Ann Oncol 2017;28(5):1137–44.

55. Wagle N, Emery C, Berger MF, et al. Dissecting therapeutic resistance to RAF inhibition in melanoma by tumor genomic profiling. J Clin Oncol 2011;29(22): 3085–96.

56. Wang AX, Qi XY. Targeting RAS/RAF/MEK/ERK signaling in metastatic melanoma. IUBMB Life 2013;65(9):748–58.

57. Yadav V, Zhang X, Liu J, et al. Reactivation of mitogen-activated protein kinase (MAPK) pathway by FGF receptor 3 (FGFR3)/Ras mediates resistance to vemurafenib in human B-RAF V600E mutant melanoma. J Biol Chem 2012;287(33): 28087–98.

58. Nazarian R, Shi H, Wang Q, et al. Melanomas acquire resistance to B-RAF(V600E) inhibition by RTK or N-RAS upregulation. Nature 2010; 468(7326):973–7.

59. Johnson DB, Puzanov I. Treatment of NRAS-mutant melanoma. Curr Treat Options Oncol 2015;16(4):15.

60. Corcoran RB, Settleman J, Engelman JA. Potential therapeutic strategies to overcome acquired resistance to BRAF or MEK inhibitors in BRAF mutant cancers. Oncotarget 2011;2(4):336–46.

61. Johnson DB, Flaherty KT, Weber JS, et al. Combined BRAF (Dabrafenib) and MEK inhibition (Trametinib) in patients with BRAFV600-mutant melanoma experiencing progression with single-agent BRAF inhibitor. J Clin Oncol 2014;32(33): 3697–704.

62. Chen G, McQuade JL, Panka DJ, et al. Clinical, molecular, and immune analysis of dabrafenib-trametinib combination treatment for BRAF inhibitor-refractory metastatic melanoma: a phase 2 clinical trial. JAMA Oncol 2016;2(8):1056–64.

63. Schreuer M, Jansen Y, Planken S, et al. Combination of dabrafenib plus trametinib for BRAF and MEK inhibitor pretreated patients with advanced BRAF(V600)-mutant melanoma: an open-label, single arm, dual-centre, phase 2 clinical trial. Lancet Oncol 2017;18(4):464–72.

64. Balch CM, Soong SJ, Smith T, et al. Long-term results of a prospective surgical trial comparing 2 cm vs. 4 cm excision margins for 740 patients with 1-4 mm melanomas. Ann Surg Oncol 2001;8(2):101–8.
65. Chen JY, Hruby G, Scolyer RA, et al. Desmoplastic neurotropic melanoma: a clinicopathologic analysis of 128 cases. Cancer 2008;113(10):2770–8.
66. Strom T, Caudell JJ, Han D, et al. Radiotherapy influences local control in patients with desmoplastic melanoma. Cancer 2014;120(9):1369–78.
67. Guadagnolo BA, Prieto V, Weber R, et al. The role of adjuvant radiotherapy in the local management of desmoplastic melanoma. Cancer 2014;120(9):1361–8.
68. ClinicalTrials.com. Neurotropic melanoma of the head and neck (RTN2). Available at: https://clinicaltrials.gov/ct2/show/NCT00975520. Accessed October 2, 2019.
69. Henderson MA, Burmeister BH, Ainslie J, et al. Adjuvant lymph-node field radiotherapy versus observation only in patients with melanoma at high risk of further lymph-node field relapse after lymphadenectomy (ANZMTG 01.02/TROG 02.01): 6-year follow-up of a phase 3, randomised controlled trial. Lancet Oncol 2015; 16(9):1049–60.
70. Agrawal S, Kane JM 3rd, Guadagnolo BA, et al. The benefits of adjuvant radiation therapy after therapeutic lymphadenectomy for clinically advanced, high-risk, lymph node-metastatic melanoma. Cancer 2009;115(24):5836–44.

Novel Targets in Melanoma

Intralesional and Combination Therapy to Manipulate the Immune Response

Alicia A. Gingrich, MD, Amanda R. Kirane, MD*

KEYWORDS

- Metastatic melanoma • Immunotherapy • Combination therapy
- Intralesional therapy • Checkpoint blockage

KEY POINTS

- Overall, intralesional therapy shows great promise in the early stages, although Talimogene Laherparepvec is currently the only US Food and Drug Administration-approved intralesional therapy for melanoma.
- At the time of publication, PV-10 and Bacillus Calmette-Guerin have moved into phase III clinical trials.
- Novel targets for therapy are gaining momentum and being actively pursued as agents for combination therapy in conjunction with checkpoint inhibitors for human cancers, including metastatic melanoma.
- Intralesional therapies and novel drug targets are being investigated for use with the checkpoint inhibitors and BRAF/MEK inhibition for tumors refractory to monotherapy, with promising preclinical results.
- Most combinations are in phase I safety or phase II efficacy stages of testing at the time of publication.

INTRODUCTION

Clinical outcomes for metastatic melanoma have been dramatically altered by recent developments in immunotherapy with checkpoint blockade and targeted strategies such as BRAF/MEK inhibition.[1,2] However, overall response to these therapies is not uniform, the majority of patients do not respond, and clinical response can be self-limited with eventual relapse.[1] Therefore, strategies to target the individual's specific tumor and immune profile to overcome resistance and elicit response are of paramount interest.

Department of Surgery, University of California Davis, 4501 X Street, Suite 3010, Sacramento, CA 95817, USA
* Corresponding author.
E-mail address: arkirane@ucdavis.edu

Surg Oncol Clin N Am 29 (2020) 467–483
https://doi.org/10.1016/j.soc.2020.02.012
1055-3207/20/© 2020 Elsevier Inc. All rights reserved.

To this end, current directions in melanoma treatment aim to leverage a combination of therapies for tumors refractory to anti-programmed death (PD)-1 monotherapy. Such approaches augment local immune cell recruitment beyond T cells to modify the tumor microenvironment, target oncogenes and downstream signaling, or inhibit byproducts required for tumor metabolism.[3–6] Local tumor-directed strategies such as radiation and intralesional therapy as well as inhibitors designed for novel targets may amplify currently used systemic agents when used in combination. Here, we summarize new classes of agents and emerging multimodal combination strategies that demonstrate significant promise in future melanoma management.

INTRALESIONAL THERAPIES

Talimogene iaherparepvec (T-VEC) is an oncolytic virus that mediates tumor regression through selective replication within and lysis of tumor cells as well as induction of systemic antitumor immunity capable of eradicating tumor at distant, uninjected sites. T-VEC is derived from herpes simplex virus type I and genetically modified to preferentially replicate in tumor cells and enhance immunity by increased (1) antigen loading of major histocompatibility class I molecules and (2) expression of granulocyte macrophage colony-stimulating factor to increase tumor-antigen presentation by dendritic cells.[3,7] Intratumoral T-VEC has been shown to be safe and is approved as intralesional therapy for patients with unresectable stage IIIB through IV melanoma.[8,9] Significant overall response rate (64% in injected lesions) and bystander effect (34% in uninjected lesions) was observed in phase III studies with minimal side effect profile.[7,10]

Mechanistically, T-VEC has been shown to increase the CD8+ T-cell infiltrate into the tumor bed, thus priming the tumor microenvironment for treatment with checkpoint inhibitors.[11] Results from a 2-year phase II trial of T-VEC as neoadjuvant therapy in resectable stage IIIB-IVM1a melanoma (NCT02211131) also demonstrate increased CD8+ cell density, which was correlated with clinical outcomes.[12] The 2- year recurrence-free survival and overall survival rates were both improved with neoadjuvant intralesional T-VEC plus surgery when compared with surgery alone.[12] T-VEC also decreases immunosuppressing regulatory T cell population and may generate long-lasting immunity, leading to durable control at uninjected sites.[3,7,11,12]

A related oncolytic virus is canerpaturev, also known as C-VEC and formerly HF10. This virus is a spontaneous mutant of herpes simplex virus 1 that preferentially replicates in tumor cells, like T-VEC.[13,14] herpes simplex virus is a focus of oncolytic research owing to its large genomic size, making it able to accommodate large transgenes, and its ability to infect a range of hosts, including common preclinical species models such as mice and monkeys.[14] Canerpaturev induces tumor cell necrosis with the increased infiltration of CD8+ T cells. Studies in a mouse model have demonstrated a release of IL-2, IL-12, interferon (IFN)-alpha, IFN-beta, IFN-gamma, and tumor necrosis facto-alpha by splenocytes when exposed to squamous cell carcinoma cells in vitro following treatment with canerpaturev. This drug has been used in phase Ib trials to treat melanoma in addition to other cutaneous head and neck cancers with good clinical success (NCT01017185).[14,15]

CAVATAK is a coxsackievirus A21-based oncolytic viral therapy also used for the intralesional treatment of melanoma.[16] This virus is very common RNA virus targeting intracellular adhesion molecule-1 (ICAM-1), which is upregulated on the surface of many cancers, including melanoma.[16] Once taken in by ICAM-1–expressing cells, the cancer cell machinery is hijacked for viral replication and eventual cell lysis. The phase II study for CAVATAK demonstrated durable response of 38.6% of patients in both injected and uninjected lesions, thereby producing the bystander effect seen in other regional therapies.[17] Follow-up extension studies showed an influx of immune cells to the tumor bed after CAVATAK injection. Additionally, digital RNA counting identified an increase in targetable checkpoint molecules, a promising finding to support combination therapy with checkpoint inhibitors.[17]

Another intralesional agent is rose Bengal disodium, a xanthene dye used in diagnostic ophthalmology and to study liver function tests.[18,19] When formulated as a 10% sterile, nonpyrogenic saline solution, it is known as PV-10, and this agent has become a focus for intralesional melanoma therapy. During preclinical testing, it was noted that lesions injected with PV-10 contained increased amounts of tumor infiltrating lymphocytes.[19] Although its precise mechanism of action is unknown, PV-10 seems to induce a systemic immune response as evidenced by local tumor destruction via lysis of tumor cells, as well as a bystander effect on uninjected lesions.[19] Phase II trials demonstrated good local control with a durable effect and complete response in 50% of patients.[18] Again, low toxicity was seen with the predominant adverse effects consisting of blistering at the treatment site. A recent propensity score-matched study demonstrated comparable survival after isolated limb infusion versus PV-10.[20]

One of the first agents to be used for intralesional injection was IL-2.[21] Initial phase II trials reported a 62.5% response rate when injected into metastatic lesions. Previously, systemic IL-2 had been used to treat metastatic melanoma, but this treatment carried significant adverse effects and toxicities.[22] More recently, intralesional IL-2 has been used in combination with topical imiquimod, because this combination is thought to restore the Th1 response (IL-2, IFN-γ, tumor necrosis factor-β) in patients with metastatic cancer, which have a predominantly Th2 response (IL-4, IL-5, IL-6, IL-10, and IL-13).[23,24] Imiquimod activates toll-like receptor 7, increasing natural killer cell activity and resulting in a robust release of cytokines to include those in the Th1 response. In clinical trials, the combination of intralesional IL-2 plus imiquimod resulted in good local control and evidence of systemic immune response, but without the toxicity of intravenous IL-2. Patients treated in this group experienced 100% clinical response rate and have demonstrated no relapse in longitudinal follow-up.[23] Ongoing trials are exploring the use of intralesional IL-2 as a fusion protein with L19, a fully human recombinant monoclonal antibody (NCT02076633, NCT01253096) and in liposomal form (NCT00004104).

A comprehensive listing of the ongoing intralesional clinical trials (early phase through phase III) for metastatic melanoma is listed in **Table 1**. Overall, intralesional therapy shows great promise in the early stages, although T-VEC is currently the only intralesional therapy approved by the US Food and Drug Administration for melanoma. At the time of publication, PV-10 and BCG have moved into phase III clinical trials.

NEW TARGETED AGENTS TO AUGMENT IMMUNOTHERAPY

An emerging group of immunotherapeutic targets present opportunities for targets for patients without BRAF mutation, or those whose tumors have developed BRAF resistance. The properties of these agents may also open the door to increased efficacy of checkpoint inhibition when used in combination to prime the immune system. These new potential targets are being studied in the context of combination therapy to complement BRAF/MEK or PD-1/PD- ligand 1 (L1) as a multifaceted manipulation of the immune system to fight metastatic disease.[1,4]

The TYRO3, AXL, and MERTK receptor tyrosine kinase family have been associated with a number of human cancers, including melanoma. Effects attributed to oncogenesis and metastasis (epithelial-to-mesenchymal transition) of the TYRO3, AXL, and

Table 1
Clinical trials of intralesional therapies for melanoma

NCT Number	Phase	Title	Interventions
NCT01209676	Early phase I	IMCgp100 in Advanced Unresectable Melanoma	IMCgp100 injection
NCT03655756	Early phase I	pDNA Intralesional Cancer Vaccine for Cutaneous Melanoma	IFx-Hu2.0
NCT01017185	Phase I	Study of HF10 in Patients With Refractory Head and Neck Cancer or Solid Tumors With Cutaneous and/or Superficial Lesions	HF10
NCT00219843	Phase I	Intralesional PV-10 Chemoablation of Metastatic Melanoma	PV-10 (rose Bengal disodium, 10%)
NCT01838200	Phase I	Phase I Study of Intralesional Bacillus Calmette-Guerin (BCG) Followed by Ipilimumab in Advanced Metastatic Melanoma	Bacillus Calmette-Guerin vaccine, ipilimumab, isoniazid
NCT03989895	Phase I	Arm 2: Intratumoral Injection of Dengue Virus-1 #45AZ5 (PV-001-DV) in Patients With Advanced Melanoma	Dengue virus-1 #45AZ5 (PV-001-DV)
NCT00815607	Phase I	Trial of an Intratumoral Injections of INXN-3001 in Subjects With Stage III or IV Melanoma	INXN-3001
NCT03747744	Phase I	Intratumoral Injection of Autologous CD1c (BDCA-1)+ Myeloid Dendritic Cells Plus Talimogene Laherparepvec (T-VEC)	CD1c (BDCA-1)+ myeloid DC + T-VEC
NCT03052205	Phase I	A Study of Intratumoral IMO-2125 in Patients With Refractory Solid Tumors	IMO-2125
NCT01123304	Phase I	Safety Study of Human IgM (MORAb-028) to Treat Metastatic Melanoma	MORAb028
NCT03803397	Phase I	Arm 1: Infusion of Autologous Monocyte-derived Lysate Pulsed Dendritic Cells (PV-001-DC) in Patients With Advanced Melanoma	PV-001-DC
NCT00003556	Phase I	Vaccine Therapy in Treating Patients With Melanoma	ALVAC-hB7.1, canarypox-hIL-12 melanoma vaccine
NCT01469455	Phase I	DNA Repair Inhibitor & Irradiation on Melanoma	DT01

(continued on next page)

Table 1 *(continued)*			
NCT Number	**Phase**	**Title**	**Interventions**
NCT00574977	Phase I	Safety Study of Modified Vaccinia Virus to Cancer	Vaccinia virus (vvDD-CDSR)
NCT02680184	Phase I	Clinical Study of CMP-001 in Combination With Pembrolizumab or as a Monotherapy	CMP-001, pembrolizumab
NCT02668770	Phase I	Ipilimumab (Immunotherapy) and MGN1703 (TLR Agonist) in Patients With Advanced Solid Malignances	MGN1703, ipilimumab
NCT00625456	Phase I	Safety Study of Recombinant Vaccinia Virus to Treat Refractory Solid Tumors	RAC VAC GM-CSF (JX-594)
NCT01935453	Phase I	A Phase I Study of Recombinant hGM-CSF Herpes Simplex Virus to Treat Cancer	Recombinant hGM-CSF herpes simplex virus injection
NCT01986426	Phase I	LTX-315 in Patients With Transdermally Accessible Tumors as Monotherapy or Combination With Ipilimumab or Pembrolizumab	LTX-315 + ipilimumab, LTX-315 + pembrolizumab
NCT02576665	Phase I	A Study of Toca 511, a Retroviral Replicating Vector, Combined With Toca FC in Patients With Solid Tumors or Lymphoma (Toca 6)	Toca 511, Toca FC
NCT02428036	Phase I	A Study of TBI-1401(HF10) in Patients With Solid Tumors With Superficial Lesions	TBI-1401 (HF10)
NCT03301896	Phase I	Study of the Safety and Efficacy of LHC165 Single Agent and in Combination With PDR001 in Patients With Advanced Malignancies	LHC165, PDR001
NCT02988960	Phase I	A Study of ABBV-927 and ABBV-181, an Immunotherapy, in Subjects With Advanced Solid Tumors	ABBV-927, ABBV-181
NCT00022568	Phase I	Vaccine Therapy in Treating Patients With Metastatic Melanoma	Recombinant vaccinia-TRICOM vaccine

(continued on next page)

Table 1
(continued)

NCT Number	Phase	Title	Interventions
NCT00004148	Phase I	Vaccine Therapy in Treating Patients With Unresectable Metastatic Melanoma	Recombinant vaccinia-B7.1 vaccine
NCT00005057	Phase I	Gene Therapy and Ganciclovir in Treating Patients With Stage IV Melanoma	Adenovirus RSV-TK, ganciclovir
NCT03712358	Phase I	PVSRIPO for Patients With Unresectable Melanoma	PVSRIPO
NCT00623831	Phase I	A Phase 1 Study of Mixed Bacteria Vaccine (MBV) in Patients With Tumors Expressing NY-ESO-1 Antigen	Mixed bacterial vaccine
NCT01082887	Phase I Phase II	A Study of Immunotherapy With TIL (Tumor Infiltrating Lymphocytes) in Combination With Intra-tumoral Injections of Interferon Gamma-adenovirus (Ad-IFNg) in Patients With Stage IIIc or Stage IV Metastatic Melanoma (AJCC)(Protocol TIL-Ad-INFg)	TIL + INFG
NCT02225366	Phase I Phase II	Intratumoral Injections of LL37 for Melanoma	LL37
NCT01397708	Phase I Phase II	Safety Study of Adenovirus Vector Engineered to Express hIL-12 in Combination With Activator Ligand to Treat Melanoma	INXN-2001
NCT00429312	Phase I Phase II	A Study of Recombinant Vaccinia Virus to Treat Malignant Melanoma	JX-594
NCT00002817	Phase I Phase II	Vaccine Therapy in Treating Patients With Metastatic Melanoma	Sargramostim, vaccinia-GM-CSF vaccine
NCT01227551	Phase II	A Study of Intratumoral CAVATAK in Patients With Stage IIIc and Stage IV Malignant Melanoma (VLA-007 CALM)	Coxsackievirus A21 (CVA21, CAVATAK)
NCT01253096	Phase II	Intratumoral Application of L19IL2 in Patients With Malignant Melanoma	L19IL2

(continued on next page)

Table 1
(continued)

NCT Number	Phase	Title	Interventions
NCT01636882	Phase II	CAVATAK in Patients With Stage IIIc or IV Malignant Melanoma to Extend Dosing to 48 Weeks (VLA-008 CALM Ext)	CVA21
NCT00521053	Phase II	Phase 2 Study of Intralesional PV-10 for Metastatic Melanoma	PV-10
NCT00204581	Phase II	Intralesional Treatment With Interleukin-2 (Proleukin) in Soft Tissue Melanoma Metastases	IL-2
NCT02076633	Phase II	Intratumoral Administration of L19IL2/L19TNF	L19IL2 + L19TNF
NCT03190824	Phase II	Evaluate Efficacy, Immunologic Response of Intratumoral/Intralesional Oncolytic Virus (OBP-301) in Metastatic Melanoma	OBP-301
NCT03754140	Phase II	Intralesional Sclerosant for in Transit and Cutaneous Melanoma Metastases	Polidocanol injection
NCT03928275	Phase II Phase III	The Response to Intralesional IL-2 and/or BCG Treatment for Cutaneous Metastatic Melanoma	Bacillus Calmette-Guerin + IL-2
NCT02288897	Phase III	PV-10 vs Chemotherapy or Oncolytic Viral Therapy for Treatment of Locally Advanced Cutaneous Melanoma	PV-10 + dacarbazine, temozolomide or talimogene laherparepvec

MERTK receptors have been described. In particular, the AXL tyrosine kinase receptor has been implicated with poorer prognosis in many human cancers, including certain resistant phenotypes of melanoma and failure to respond to targeted therapy or checkpoint blockade.[25–27] Similar to immune checkpoint, AXL serves as a negative immune regulator in response to inflammation and injury, a mechanism that is highjacked in the tumor setting to promote unchecked growth.[25–30] AXL receptor function significantly manipulates epithelial to mesenchymal plasticity in the tumor microenvironment, influencing ligand secretion by macrophages. This finding has been correlated in preclinical in vivo studies with significant increase in metastatic potential for AXL-expressing tumors, with metastatic events eliminated by multiple strategies of AXL inhibition. Response was greatest in immunocompetent models, highlighting the interplay between this pathway and immune cell function.[31] The interaction of AXL with various cellular process is illustrated in **Fig. 1**.[27]

The AXL pathway may critically contribute to adaptive or evasive immune resistance because it is seen to be significantly activated in chemotherapy resistant breast and

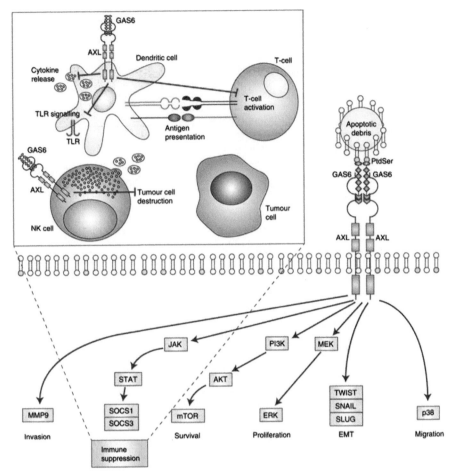

Fig. 1. Spectrum of cellular processes regulated by AXL activity. AXL, after activation by its ligand growth arrest-specific 6 along with an interaction between growth arrest-specific 6 and phosphatidylserine (PtdSer), dimerises and cross-phosphorylates (*yellow circle*) its partner receptor. This activation regulates an array of cellular pathways as illustrated at the bottom of the figure. *Inset*: AXL activity plays a complex role in immune regulation that includes the inhibition of cytokine release, toll-like receptor signaling, and T-cell activation by antigen-presenting cells such as dendritic cells (above), as well as specific antitumor killing by natural killer cells (below). (*From* Gay, C.M., K. Balaji, and L.A. Byers, *Giving AXL the axe: targeting AXL in human malignancy.* British Journal of Cancer, 2017. 116(4): p. 415; with permission.)

pancreatic models as well as radioinsensitive melanoma.[25,27] Early preclinical data demonstrates Axl ligand, growth arrest-specific 6 influences suppressive function of regulatory T cells and inhibits natural killer and dendritic cell maturation, thereby dampening antitumor immune response.[28,30,32,33] Axl expression has been shown to predict checkpoint blockage failure in melanoma patients.[26] Preclinical models investigating Axl-inhibition in combination with PD-1 demonstrated a synergistic effect evidenced by unregulated PD-L1 expression.[31] Mechanistic studies unveiled that Axl inhibition increased the proliferation of CD8[+] T cells, likely through dendritic cells and the activation of CD103[+] during cross-presentation.[31] Anti-Axl is being investigated with the drug TP-0903 (NCT02729298) to treat all solid tumors, including melanoma. A second anti-Axl small molecule inhibitor, bemcentinib, has recently shown efficacy in a phase II trial (NCT03184571) for lung adenocarcinoma in patients with low/no PD-1 expression. Moreover, the combination of bemcentinib and pembrolizumab was well-tolerated.[34]

Indoleamine 2,3-dioxygenase (IDO), an immunomodulatory enzyme is produced by myeloid-derived suppressor cells and inhibits the immune response by depletion of the amino acid tryptophan, thereby affecting tumor metabolism and altering the tumor microenvironment type.[35] IDO contributes to immune suppression and tolerance by suppressing the proliferation and differentiation of effector T cells, and enhancing the activity of regulatory T cells.[36,37] In the absence of tumor, IDO is systemically required for tolerance. This enzyme is found in the gut and on mucosal surfaces, and IDO-deficient mice have been shown to reject their fetuses. IDO works by direct suppression of proinflammatory TH17 cytokines IL-6 and IL-17. However, in the setting of cancer, this natural promotion of immune tolerance is hijacked by tumors and leads to unchecked tumor growth. In immunogenically cold lesions, the inhibition of IDO could prevent immune tolerance and allow for robust immune response when followed by the administration of intralesional oncolytic virus.[36,37] In a companion canine model of metastatic melanoma and sarcoma, systemic IDO inhibition was found to augment response to local treatment with radiotherapy with good efficacy and limited toxicity.[38] Anti-IDO is being investigated as DX-03-12 and DX-03-13 (NCT03047928) used in combination nivolumab and PD-L1/IDO peptide vaccine. A separate trial, NCT04007588, uses BMS-986205 as the anti-IDO drug in the presence and absence of both nivolumab and ipilimumab.

Efficiency of the T-cell response is paramount to harnessing the immune system for tumor eradication. Certain T-cell markers, among them TIGIT and LAG3, have been found to represent an exhausted phenotype of T cells, characterized by decreased cytotoxicity and effector function.[39,40] Lymphocyte activating gene, in particular, is expressed on CD4+ and CD8+ T cells and has been shown to act in synergy with PD-1 to downregulate T cells. It is thought that the lymphocyte activating gene operates through preventing calcium influx via T-cell receptors, which downstream leads to decreased expansion and eventual reduction in the amount of memory T cells. Evidence of enriched coexpression of lymphocyte activating gene and PD-1 was seen on tumor infiltrating lymphocytes in ovarian cancer.[40] A second method to circumvent T-cell exhaustion lies in the interaction between T-cell Ig and ITIM domain (TIGIT), which is expressed by tumor infiltrating lymphocytes, and CD155, which is expressed by tumor cells, and in particular melanomas.[39] TIGIT expression is noted to be highest on CD8+ T cells. When bound by the inhibitory CD155, this induces inhibition of the classic CD8+ T-cell effector function and allows the tumor to evade immune response.[39] Anti-LAG3 is being investigated as adjuvant therapy with nivolumab and pembrolizumab (NCT02676869, NCT03743766) and in a separate trial with nivolumab and ipilimumab (NCT02519322). The anti-TIGIT drug BGB-A1217 has an ongoing study with tislelizumab (and anti-PD1 agent) in advanced solid tumors (NCT04047862). A recent study of anti-TIGIT plus nivolumab was terminated (NCT03119428).

INTRALESIONAL AND SYSTEMIC COMBINATION THERAPIES

As is well-known, the response rate for checkpoint inhibition and intralesional therapy is not universal. Although it has long been accepted that a tumor's genetic mutational burden drives its biologic behavior, there is a growing appreciation for the role of the immune phenotype of the tumor to predict and dictate response to treatment, particularly immunotherapy. Hot tumors are have high immunologic infiltrate, whereas cold tumors are non–T-cell inflamed cancers.[41,42] Hot tumors have higher expression of T-cell markers, IFN, IDO, and PD-1, to name a few, and thus are more responsive to immunotherapy. Naturally, the next steps involve questions of how we may manipulate the immune phenotype of tumors to elicit a greater pathologic response. To this end, combination therapy leveraging intralesional therapies and systemic therapies is being explored (**Table 2**).

The combination of T-VEC plus anti–PD-1 therapy was first investigated by Ribas, and colleagues[11] Intratumoral injection with T-VEC resulted in an influx of CD8$^+$ T cells into the tumor, increased PD-L1 protein expression, and induced IFN-γ gene expression. When T-VEC was administered in combination with ipilimumab, a synergistic effect was seen as evidenced by improved efficacy. Importantly, as seen in their phase Ib trial, this effect did not occur in the setting of increased toxicity.[8,11] The phase III follow-on study, MASTERKEY-265, is currently active with 713 participants to evaluate T-VEC plus pembrolizumab when compared with placebo injection plus pembrolizumab for 24 months from the date of first treatment or disappearance of lesions (NCT02263508).

Canerpaturev (HF10) has been tested in phase II trials in combination with ipilimumab for patients with unresectable/unresected stage IIIB to IV melanoma (NCT02272855). This combination demonstrated a median progression-free survival of 19 months and a median overall survival of 26 months.[43,44] Molecular studies of the tumors revealed increased CD8$^+$ T-cell infiltrate and decreased CD4$^+$ T cells.[43] In this study, 28.3% of patients had grade 3 or higher adverse events, most which were attributed to ipilimumab and only 3 attributed to intralesional therapy.[43]

Combination therapy has been studied using CAVATAK and PD-1 blockade in an immune competent murine model using B16-ICAM-1 melanoma.[45] Authors in this study noted greater antitumor activity of the CAVATAK plus PD-1 monoclonal antibody when compared with saline controls. Although this method does rely on the expression of ICAM-I by the tumor cells, a survival benefit was seen in the mice. Based on this preclinical evidence, phase I trials combining CAVATAK with either pembrolizumab (NCT02565992) or ipilimumab (NCT02307149) have been initiated in the United States.[46] A second preclinical trial in immune competent mice was conducted to study CAVATAK in addition to PD-1 blockade and anti-IDO. CAVATAK plus anti-IDO alone was not associated with a significant reduction in tumor size, but triple therapy was superior to CAVATAK plus PD-1 blockade alone.[47]

A completed phase I trial examined the response of intratumoral IL-2 and intratumoral ipilimumab in 12 patients (NCT01672450). Because the systemic checkpoint inhibitors are not without side effects, it was postulated that intralesional injections of each agent would decrease systemic toxicity. Overall, the local response to therapy was 67% and a bystander response was seen in 89%.[48] There were no dose-limiting toxicities and all patients completed treatment. A separate phase II trial examined intralesional IL-2 with systemic ipilimumab (NCT01480323). The overall efficacy rate in this study was 20%, with 40% of patients experiencing a grade III/IV adverse event.[49] The results ultimately suggested that the combination therapy did not show improved efficacy over ipilimumab alone.

An international phase Ib/II study is currently underway to determine the safety and efficacy of PV-10 in combination with pembrolizumab (NCT02557321). Patients with metastatic melanoma will receive either PV-10 plus pembrolizumab or pembrolizumab alone. There are no data available as of yet, because the primary study completion date is anticipated to occur in April 2020. Before this trial, a small, 3-person case series

Table 2
Clinical trials of combinations with intralesional and checkpoint therapies

NCT Number	Phase	Title	Interventions
NCT01672450	Phase I	A Study of Intratumoral Injection of Interleukin-2 and Ipilimumab in Patients With Unresectable Stages III-IV Melanoma	Intratumoral ipilimumab and IL-2
NCT02565992	Phase I	Intratumoral CAVATAK (CVA21) and Pembrolizumab in Patients With Advanced Melanoma (VLA-011 CAPRA)	CAVATAK + pembrolizumab
NCT02307149	Phase I	Intratumoral CAVATAK (CVA21) and Ipilimumab in Patients With Advanced Melanoma (VLA-013 MITCI)	CAVATAK + ipilimumab
NCT03291002	Phase I	Study of Intratumoral CV8102 in cMEL, cSCC, hnSCC, and ACC	CV8102 + anti-PD-1 therapy
NCT03773744	Phase I	MG1-MAGEA3 With Ad-MAGEA3 and Pembrolizumab in Patients With Previously Treated Metastatic Melanoma or Cutaneous Squamous Cell Carcinoma	Ad-MAGEA3, MG1-MAGEA3, pembrolizumab, cyclophosphamide
NCT03084640	Phase I	Phase 1B Study Evaluating Alternative Routes of Administration of CMP-001 in Combination With Pembrolizumab in Participants With Advanced Melanoma	CMP-001, pembrolizumab
NCT02680184	Phase I	Clinical Study of CMP-001 in Combination With Pembrolizumab or as a Monotherapy	CMP-001, pembrolizumab
NCT02668770	Phase I	Ipilimumab (Immunotherapy) and MGN1703 (TLR Agonist) in Patients With Advanced Solid Malignancies	MGN1703, ipilimumab
NCT01986426	Phase I	LTX-315 in Patients With Transdermally Accessible Tumors as Monotherapy or Combination With Ipilimumab or Pembrolizumab	LTX-315 + ipilimumab, LTX-315 + pembrolizumab
NCT01838200	Phase I	Phase I Study of Intralesional Bacillus Calmette-Guerin (BCG) Followed by Ipilimumab in Advanced Metastatic Melanoma	Bacillus Calmette-Guerin vaccine, ipilimumab, Isoniazid

(continued on next page)

Table 2
(continued)

NCT Number	Phase	Title	Interventions
NCT02557321	Phase I Phase II	PV-10 in Combination With Pembrolizumab for Treatment of Metastatic Melanoma	PV-10, pembrolizumab
NCT03474497	Phase I Phase II	UCDCC#272: IL-2, Radiotherapy, and Pembrolizumab in Patients Refractory to Checkpoint Blockade	IL-2, pembrolizumab, radiotherapy
NCT02719015	Phase I Phase II	Dose Escalation and Cohort Expansion of Safety and Tolerability Study of Intratumoral rAd.CD40L (ISF35) in Combination of Systemic Pembrolizumab in Patients With Refractory Metastatic Melanoma	rAd.CD40L, pembrolizumab
NCT02644967	Phase I Phase II	A Study to Assess the Safety and Efficacy of Intratumoral IMO-2125 in Combination With Ipilimumab or Pembrolizumab in Patients With Metastatic Melanoma	IMO-2125, ipilimumab, pembrolizumab
NCT02521870	Phase I Phase II	A Trial of Intratumoral Injections of SD-101 in Combination With Pembrolizumab in Patients With Metastatic Melanoma or Recurrent or Metastatic Head and Neck Squamous Cell Carcinoma	SD-101(1), pembrolizumab
NCT03958383	Phase I Phase II	IT-hu14.18-IL2 With Radiation, Nivolumab and Ipilimumab for Melanoma	hu14.18-IL2, radiation, nivolumab, ipilimumab
NCT02706353	Phase I Phase II	APX005M in Combination With Systemic Pembrolizumab in Patients With Metastatic Melanoma	APX005M, pembrolizumab
NCT03684785	Phase I Phase II	Intratumoral AST-008 Combined With Pembrolizumab in Patients With Advanced Solid Tumors	AST-008 + pembrolizumab
NCT03058289	Phase I Phase II	A Phase 1/2 Safety Study of Intratumorally Dosed INT230–6	INT230–6, anti–PD-1 antibody, anti–CTLA-4 antibody
NCT03767348	Phase I Phase II	Study of RP1 Monotherapy and RP1 in Combination With Nivolumab	RP1, nivolumab

(continued on next page)

Table 2 *(continued)*			
NCT Number	**Phase**	**Title**	**Interventions**
NCT03435640	Phase I Phase II	A Study of NKTR-262 in Combination With NKTR-214 and With NKTR-214 Plus Nivolumab in Patients With Locally Advanced or Metastatic Solid Tumor Malignancies	NKTR-262, bempegaldesleukin, nivolumab
NCT03058289	Phase I Phase II	A Phase 1/2 Safety Study of Intratumorally Dosed INT230–6	INT230-6, anti–PD-1 antibody, anti–CTLA-4 antibody
NCT01480323	Phase II	A Phase II Study to Evaluate Safety and Efficacy of Combined Treatment With Ipilimumab and Intratumoral Interleukin-2	IL-2 + ipilimumab
NCT03259425	Phase II	Neoadjuvant Trial of Nivolumab in Combination With HF10 Oncolytic Viral Therapy in Resectable Stage IIIB, IIIC, IVM1a Melanoma	Nivolumab, HF10
NCT02272855	Phase II	A Study of Combination Treatment With HF10 and Ipilimumab in Patients With Unresectable or Metastatic Melanoma	HF10, ipilimumab
NCT03132675	Phase II	Tavo and Pembrolizumab in Patients With Stage III/IV Melanoma Progressing on Pembrolizumab or Nivolumab Treatment	Tavokinogene telseplasmid, pembrolizumab
NCT02493361	Phase II	Trial of pIL-12/MK-3475 in Metastatic Melanoma	Pembrolizumab + pIL-12
NCT03153085	Phase II	A Study of Combination With TBI-1401(HF10) and Ipilimumab in Japanese Patients With Unresectable or Metastatic Melanoma	TBI-1401(HF10), ipilimumab
NCT03618641	Phase II	CMP-001 in Combo With Nivolumab in Stage IIIB/C/D Melanoma Patients With Clinically Apparent Lymph Node Disease	CMP-001, nivolumab
NCT04093323	Phase II	Polarized Dendritic Cell (aDC1) Vaccine, Interferon Alpha-2, Rintalolimid, and Celecoxib for the Treatment of HLA-A2+ Refractory Melanoma	Alpha-type-1 polarized dendritic cells, celecoxib, PD-1 ligand inhibitor, PD1 inhibitor, recombinant interferon alfa-2b, rintatolimod

(continued on next page)

Table 2 (continued)			
NCT Number	Phase	Title	Interventions
NCT03445533	Phase III	A Study of IMO-2125 in Combination With Ipilimumab vs Ipilimumab Alone in Subjects With Anti-PD-1 Refractory Melanoma (ILLUMINATE-301)	Ipilimumab, IMO-2125

was performed to describe the effects of PV-10 plus radiation therapy to the injected lesion.[50] This regimen was well-tolerated with no significant adverse events, but not validated in a follow-on controlled trial.

SUMMARY

In summary, research surrounding intralesional therapy, novel molecular targets and combination therapy is a dynamic and promising direction for melanoma research based on preclinical and early clinical evidence. In the near future, we may see utilization of such agents and combinations more readily in the clinical setting, with the potential to benefit a larger scope of patients beyond current available therapies. These trials are actively changing the landscape of surgical approach to locally advanced and metastatic melanoma and will be important in the surgical armamentarium as neoadjuvant therapies become more standard.

DISCLOSURE

The authors of this article have no commercial or financial interests to disclose.

REFERENCES

1. Ascierto PA, et al. Perspectives in melanoma: meeting report from the Melanoma Bridge (November 29th-1 December 1st, 2018, Naples, Italy). J Transl Med 2019; 17(1):234.
2. Ascierto PA, Flaherty K, Goff S. Emerging strategies in systemic therapy for the treatment of melanoma. Am Soc Clin Oncol Educ Book 2018;38:751–8.
3. Fu LQ, et al. Recent advances in oncolytic virus-based cancer therapy. Virus Res 2019;270:197675.
4. Hu-Lieskovan S, Ribas A. New combination strategies using programmed cell death 1/programmed cell death ligand 1 checkpoint inhibitors as a backbone. Cancer J 2017;23(1):10–22.
5. Khair DO, et al. Combining immune checkpoint inhibitors: established and emerging targets and strategies to improve outcomes in melanoma. Front Immunol 2019;10:453.
6. Mandala M, et al. Rationale for new checkpoint inhibitor combinations in melanoma therapy. Am J Clin Dermatol 2017;18(5):597–611.
7. Andtbacka RH. The role of talimogene laherparepvec (T-VEC) in the age of checkpoint inhibitors. Clin Adv Hematol Oncol 2016;14(8):576.
8. Puzanov I, et al. Talimogene laherparepvec in combination with ipilimumab in previously untreated, unresectable stage IIIB-IV melanoma. J Clin Oncol 2016; 34(22):2619–26.

9. Sun L, et al. Talimogene laherparepvec combined with anti-PD-1 based immunotherapy for unresectable stage III-IV melanoma: a case series. J Immunother Cancer 2018;6(1):36.

10. Cochran AJ, et al. Is sentinel node susceptibility to metastases related to nodal immune modulation? Cancer J 2015;21(1):39–46.

11. Ribas A, et al. Oncolytic virotherapy promotes intratumoral T cell infiltration and improves anti-PD-1 immunotherapy. Cell 2017;170(6):1109–19.e10.

12. Dummer R, Gyorki DE, Hyngstom J, et al. Primary 2-year results of the Phase 2, multicenter, randomized, open-label trial of efficacy and safety for talimogene laherparepvec (T-VEC) neoadjuvant treatment plus surgery vs surgery in patients with resectable stage IIIb-IVM1a melanoma. (Abstract). ESMO Conference 2019, Barcelona, Spain, 2019.

13. Yokota K, et al. 1365P final results from phase II of combination with canerpaturev (formerly HF10), an oncolytic viral immunotherapy, and ipilimumab in unresectable or metastatic melanoma in second-or later line treatment. Ann Oncol 2019;30(Supplement_5):mdz255, 053.

14. Esaki S, Goshima F, Ozaki H, et al. Oncolytic activity of HF10 in head and neck squamous cell carcinomas. Cancer Gene Ther 2019;1–14. https://doi.org/10.1038/s41417-019-0129-3.

15. Ferris RL, et al. Phase I trial of intratumoral therapy using HF10, an oncolytic HSV-1, demonstrates safety in HSV+/HSV- patients with refractory and superficial cancers. J Clin Oncol 2014;32(15_suppl):6082.

16. Andtbacka RH, Shafren DR, Grose M, et al. CAVATAK-mediated oncolytic immunotherapy in advanced melanoma patients (abstract). San Diego, CA: American Association for Cancer Research Meeting 2014; 2014.

17. Andtbacka RH, Curti BD, Hallmeyer S, et al. Phase II calm extension study: coxsackievirus A21 delivered intratumorally to patients with advanced melanoma induces immune-cell infiltration in the tumor microenvironment. J Immunother Cancer 2015;3(Suppl 2).

18. Thompson JF, et al. Phase 2 study of intralesional PV-10 in refractory metastatic melanoma. Ann Surg Oncol 2015;22(7):2135–42.

19. Ross MI. Intralesional therapy with PV 10 (Rose Bengal) for in transit melanoma. J Surg Oncol 2014;109(4):314–9.

20. Read T, et al. Patients with in-transit melanoma metastases have comparable survival outcomes following isolated limb infusion or intralesional PV-10—A propensity score matched, single center study. J Surg Oncol 2019;119(6):717–27.

21. Radny P, et al. Phase II trial of intralesional therapy with interleukin-2 in soft-tissue melanoma metastases. Br J Cancer 2003;89(9):1620.

22. Phan GQ, et al. Factors associated with response to high-dose interleukin-2 in patients with metastatic melanoma. J Clin Oncol 2001;19(15):3477–82.

23. Green D, et al. Topical imiquimod and intralesional interleukin-2 increase activated lymphocytes and restore the Th1/Th2 balance in patients with metastatic melanoma. Br J Dermatol 2008;159(3):606–14.

24. Garcia MS, et al. Complete regression of subcutaneous and cutaneous metastatic melanoma with high-dose intralesional interleukin 2 in combination with topical imiquimod and retinoid cream. Melanoma Res 2011;21(3):235–43.

25. Akalu YT, Rothlin CV, Ghosh S. TAM receptor tyrosine kinases as emerging targets of innate immune checkpoint blockade for cancer therapy. Immunol Rev 2017;276(1):165–77.

26. Davidsen KT, Haaland GS, Lie MK, et al. The role of Axl receptor tyrosine kinase in tumor cell plasticity and therapy resistance. In: Akslen, Lars A, Watnick,

editors. Biomarkers of the tumor microenvironment. New York City, NY: Springer, Cham; 2017. p. 351–76.

27. Gay CM, Balaji K, Byers LA. Giving AXL the axe: targeting AXL in human malignancy. Br J Cancer 2017;116(4):415.

28. Kim E-M, et al. Axl signaling induces development of natural killer cells in vitro and in vivo. Protoplasma 2017;254(2):1091–101.

29. Kirane A, et al. Warfarin blocks Gas6-mediated Axl activation required for pancreatic cancer epithelial plasticity and metastasis. Cancer Res 2015;75(18): 3699–705.

30. Park I-K, et al. The Axl/Gas6 pathway is required for optimal cytokine signaling during human natural killer cell development. Blood 2009;113(11):2470–7.

31. Guo Z, et al. Axl inhibition induces the antitumor immune response which can be further potentiated by PD-1 blockade in the mouse cancer models. Oncotarget 2017;8(52):89761–74.

32. Park IK, et al. A xl/G as6 pathway positively regulates FLT3 activation in human natural killer cell development. Eur J Immunol 2013;43(10):2750–5.

33. Zhao GJ, Zheng JY, Bian JL, et al. Growth arrest-specific 6 enhances the suppressive function of $CD4^+CD25^+$ regulatory T cells mainly through Axl receptor. Mediators Inflamm 2017;2017:6848430.

34. Krebs MG. NCT03184571: phase II clinical trial of selective AXL inhibitor bemcentinib in combination with pembrolizumab. SITC 34th Annual Meeting; Concurrent Session 206: High Impact Clinical Trials; Presenter: Matthew G. Krebs, MD, PhD – The University of Manchester; Date: November 8, 2019. Washington, D.C.

35. Gide TN, et al. Inter- and intrapatient heterogeneity of indoleamine 2,3-dioxygenase expression in primary and metastatic melanoma cells and the tumour microenvironment. Histopathology 2019;74(6):817–28.

36. Munn DH. Blocking IDO activity to enhance anti-tumor immunity. Front Biosci (Elite Ed) 2012;4:734–45.

37. Wen H, et al. Design and synthesis of indoleamine 2,3-dioxygenase 1 inhibitors and evaluation of their use as anti-tumor agents. Molecules 2019;24(11) [pii: E2124].

38. Monjazeb AM, et al. Blocking indolamine-2, 3-dioxygenase rebound immune suppression boosts antitumor effects of radio-immunotherapy in murine models and spontaneous canine malignancies. Clin Cancer Res 2016;22(17):4328–40.

39. Mahnke K, Enk AH. TIGIT-CD155 interactions in melanoma: a novel co-inhibitory pathway with potential for clinical intervention. J Invest Dermatol 2016; 136(1):9–11.

40. Matsuzaki J, et al. Tumor-infiltrating NY-ESO-1–specific CD8+ T cells are negatively regulated by LAG-3 and PD-1 in human ovarian cancer. Proc Natl Acad Sci U S A 2010;107(17):7875–80.

41. Gajewski TF, Corrales L, William J, et al. Cancer immunotherapy targets based on understanding the T cell-inflamed versus non-T cell-inflamed tumor microenvironment. In: Kalinski, Pawel, editors. Tumor immune microenvironment in cancer progression and cancer therapy. New York City, NY: Springer, Cham; 2017. p. 19–31.

42. Maleki Vareki S. High and low mutational burden tumors versus immunologically hot and cold tumors and response to immune checkpoint inhibitors. J Immunother Cancer 2018;6(1):157.

43. Andtbacka RHI, et al. Efficacy and genetic analysis for a phase II multicenter trial of HF10, a replication-competent HSV-1 oncolytic immunotherapy, and ipilimumab combination treatment in patients with stage IIIb-IV unresectable or metastatic melanoma. J Clin Oncol 2018;36(15_suppl):9541.

44. Andtbacka RHI, et al. Final results of a phase II multicenter trial of HF10, a replication-competent HSV-1 oncolytic virus, and ipilimumab combination treatment in patients with stage IIIB-IV unresectable or metastatic melanoma. J Clin Oncol 2017;35(15_suppl):9510.

45. Shafren D, et al. Combination of a novel oncolytic immunotherapeutic agent, CAV-ATAK (coxsackievirus A21) and immune-checkpoint blockade significantly reduces tumor growth and improves survival in an immune competent mouse melanoma model. J Immunother Cancer 2014;2(3):P125.

46. Curti BD, et al. Activity of a novel immunotherapy combination of intralesional Coxsackievirus A21 and systemic ipilimumab in advanced melanoma patients previously treated with anti-PD1 blockade therapy. J Clin Oncol 2017; 35(15_suppl):3014.

47. Yuan M, Wong Y, Shafren D, et al. Pre-clinical activity of a novel immunotherapy combination of CAVATAK (Coxsackie virus A21), anti-PD-1 blockade and an IDO inhibitor in melanoma (abstract). Society for Immunotherapy of Cancer Annual Meeting 2017. Washington, D.C. 2017.

48. Ray A, et al. A phase I study of intratumoral ipilimumab and interleukin-2 in patients with advanced melanoma. Oncotarget 2016;7(39):64390-9.

49. Weide B, et al. Combined treatment with ipilimumab and intratumoral interleukin-2 in pretreated patients with stage IV melanoma—safety and efficacy in a phase II study. Cancer Immunol Immunother 2017;66(4):441-9.

50. Foote MC, et al. A novel treatment for metastatic melanoma with intralesional rose Bengal and radiotherapy: a case series. Melanoma Res 2010;20(1):48-51.

Role of Surgery in Stage IV Melanoma

Conor H. O'Neill, MD, Kelly M. McMasters, MD, PhD, Michael E. Egger, MD, MPH*

KEYWORDS

- Melanoma • Cutaneous malignancy • Metastasectomy • Stage IV melanoma
- Metastatic melanoma

KEY POINTS

- Historically, stage IV melanoma carried a poor prognosis and surgery was the only potential for cure.
- New targeted therapies, systemic immune therapies, and oncolytic viruses have achieved durable responses in advanced melanoma.
- In the era of modern systemic therapy, metastasectomy can be associated with good long-term survival.
- With effective targeted and systemic therapy, response to treatment helps appropriately selected patients who would likely benefit from metastasectomy.

INTRODUCTION

Melanoma remains the most fatal form of skin cancer and will account for more than 7000 estimated deaths in 2019.[1] Most melanomas are early stage and remain highly treatable, but up to 4% of patients present with stage IV disease and 20% of surgically treated patients will develop distant recurrences.[2,3] Historically, patients with stage IV disease have had poor overall survival, with an estimated 5-year survival rate of 6% and a median survival of less than 1 year.[4]

Metastasectomy historically has been associated with modest outcomes at best, owing to the inherent aggressive underlying biology and lack of effective systemic therapy.[5,6] The median disease-free interval (DFI) after metastasectomy for stage IV melanoma was 8 months in the era before effective systemic therapy.[6] Outcomes for resection of metastatic melanoma depended on the location and volume of the metastases. In very well-selected patients, metastasectomy was associated with a 5-year overall survival rate of 22% for patients with M1a disease consisting of subcutaneous metastases.[5] The 5-year survival rate after resection of lung metastasis was

The Hiram C. Polk Jr., MD, Department of Surgery, University of Louisville, 315 East Broadway, M-10, Louisville, KY 40202, USA
* Corresponding author. Department of Surgery, Division of Surgical Oncology, 315 E Broadway, M-10, Louisville, KY 40202.
E-mail address: michael.egger@louisville.edu

Surg Oncol Clin N Am 29 (2020) 485–495
https://doi.org/10.1016/j.soc.2020.02.010

14% in the era before high-quality cross-sectional imaging.[5] The Southwest Oncology Group intergroup trial (S9430) of resection of stage IV melanoma for multiple sites of metastases reported a 4-year overall survival of 29%.[7] Recent data have shown improvements in outcome. The MMAIT-IV trial analysis compared adjuvant Bacillus Calmette-Guérin and Canvaxin to Bacillus Calmette-Guérin (+) placebo for metastatic patients who underwent complete resection of up to 5 metastatic lesions. No improvements in survival were seen with this adjuvant therapy; however, it was noted that placebo patients attained a 60.6-month median overall survival for M1a disease, a 37.6% 5-year overall survival after lung metastasectomy, and a 5-year overall survival of 43% among all groups after metastasectomy.[8] Certainly, the 5-year survival rate for highly selected patients can be improved with metastasectomy.[5,9,10]

Improvement in outcomes for operative resection of metastatic melanoma have been achieved not from improvements in surgery, but rather from improvements in systemic therapy. Before the widespread availability of effective immunotherapy, operative resection in highly selected patients with limited metastatic disease was probably more effective than the therapeutic agents in use at the time. Data from the Multicenter Selective Lymphadenectomy Trial-1 (MSLT-1) showed metastasectomy was associated with improvement in 4-year survival to 21% versus 7% for systemic medical therapy alone.[3,11] Systemic medical therapy at that time largely consisted of dacarbazine or other cytotoxic chemotherapy drugs, either alone or in combination. Some patients with excellent performance status received high-dose IL-2 or biochemotherapy (regimens containing ≥ 1 cytotoxic agent along with IL-2 and interferon) with limited response rates and high toxicity. The treatment of metastatic melanoma, and the role of surgical resection, would evolve as the systemic therapies evolved. Currently, both BRAF/MEK inhibitors and immune checkpoint inhibitor therapies have improved survival and led to high response rates. Immunotherapy provides reasonable durable complete response rates, whereas BRAF/MEK inhibitors have very high response rates that are less durable.[12,13] Importantly, not all patients respond to therapy and not all responses are durable,[14] raising new questions regarding the appropriate role of surgery for stage IV disease.

- Metastasectomy can offer improvements in overall survival in highly selected patients.

EVOLUTION OF THERAPY

Dacarbazine, an alkylating agent, was the principle cytotoxic systemic agent historically used for the treatment of melanoma. Response rates were at best 20% and the majority of responses were partial, with fewer than 5% complete responses.[15,16] Combination therapy, such as the multiagent Dartmouth regimen (dacarbazine, cisplatin, 1.3-bis[2-chloroethyl]-1-nitrosourea, and tamoxifen) did not show any improvement over dacarbazine alone.[17] To date, there is no convincing evidence that cytotoxic chemotherapy improves overall survival in melanoma.

Improvements in response rates were ultimately demonstrated with the transition to immune-modulating agents. High-dose IL-2, a proinflammatory cytokine that activates lymphocytes, had response rates similar to cytotoxic chemotherapy on the order of 15% to 20%, but strikingly 40% of responders demonstrated durable response beyond 5 years.[18] Other agents, including Interferon-α2b and pegylated interferon- α, were of more limited benefit.[19–22]

Immune checkpoint inhibitor therapy became the first modality to demonstrate promising improvements in overall survival. Ipilimumab, a cytotoxic T-lymphocyte-associated antigen 4 inhibitor, improved median overall survival to 10.1 months in stage IV malignant melanoma.[23] Newer agents targeting the programmed death protein-1 molecule, such as nivolumab, demonstrated improved adverse event profiles compared with ipilimumab, with durable objective responses approaching 40% and the 12-month recurrence-free survival of 70.5% versus 60.8% with ipilimumab.[24–26] These response rates were further improved with combination cytotoxic T-lymphocyte-associated antigen-4 and pro-grammed death-1 therapy; objective responses were 61% in combination nivolumab and ipilimumab therapy versus 11% with monotherapy ipilimumab.[12] This effect is not without a high incidence (54%) of grade 3 or 4 toxicity.

Targeted therapies to BRAF V600 mutant melanomas, which are present in at least 40% of cutaneous melanomas, have shown an overall response rate of 48% in patients with stage IV disease, whereas combination BRAF inhibition with a MEK inhibitor such as trametinib may improve the overall response rate to 68% to 87%.[27–30] Despite an excellent objective response, the duration of response is limited and the median progression free survival is 5.1 months for BRAF inhibitor monotherapy.[31]

Talimogene laherparepvec (T-VEC) is an oncolytic virus expressing granulocyte-macrophage colony-stimulating factor derived from type 1 herpes simplex virus.[32] This process leads to the release of tumor-specific antigens and expression of granulocyte-macrophage colony-stimulating factor, which has been shown to activate T cells for an antitumor response and induce dendritic cell maturation.[33] T-VEC has been modified to selectively replicate within tumor cells, leading to tumor cell lysis and immune cell recruitment.[34,35]

T-VEC oncolytic immunotherapy was first trialed in patients with unresectable stage IIIb or IV melanoma and provided a durable response rate of 16.3% (95% confidence interval, 12.1%–20.5%).[36] Several studies have evaluated T-VEC alone or in combina-tion with systemic immunotherapy and have shown promising results with an overall response rate approaching 50% and an 18-month overall survival rate of 67%.[32,37,38] Oncolytic virotherapy with T-VEC provides an additional strategy for treatment of patients with advanced melanoma.

Before the advent of effective treatments for advanced melanoma, surgical resection was considered the standard-of-care treatment for resectable stage IV disease. However, the advent of modern melanoma therapy has ushered in a whole new set of questions regarding the most appropriate role of surgery for metastatic melanoma.

- Early systemic therapies were largely toxic with low response rates.
- BRAF/MEK inhibition has shown objective response rates in 68% to 87% of pa-tients, and durable objective responses have been found with immunotherapy.
- These improvements alter the landscape for the role of surgery in metastatic melanoma.

METASTASECTOMY

Metastasectomy, or operative resection of metastatic disease, may play an important role in the multidisciplinary, comprehensive treatment plan for patients with stage IV melanoma. Some, but not all, patients may benefit from surgery to render them dis-ease free. In some cases, metastasectomy may result in durable recurrence-free sur-vival. However, many factors must be considered when selecting patients for resection of metastatic melanoma. A true multidisciplinary discussion must be held to consider the timing of surgery in relation to systemic therapy and the goals of oper-ative resection.

Prognostic Factors to Select Suitability for Resection

An evaluation of the extent of metastatic disease is essential. Patients with a new diagnosis of metastatic melanoma, whether they present with metastatic disease at initial presentation or they develop metastatic disease as a recurrence, should be thoroughly investigated by high-resolution cross-sectional imaging of the chest, abdomen and pelvis either by computed tomography scan or PET/computed tomography scan and brain MRI.[39] High-quality imaging can detect early, otherwise clinically inapparent resectable metastatic disease and provide a baseline for evaluation of response to therapy. The full extent of disease is an important consideration for treatment planning purposes.

The ideal candidates for metastasectomy have a single site of metastasis and a long DFI before metastasis.[40,41] Overall survival is better for patients with a limited number of metastatic sites. In an early, preimmunotherapy study, patients who underwent metastasectomy for a single metastatic tumor had a 5-year survival rate of 29%, compared with a 5-year survival rate of 11% for those with 4 metastatic sites.[40] The DFI has been shown to predict survival. Patients who present with metastases within 1 year from the initial diagnosis have a worse outcome than those who present with a longer DFI.[42] Collectively, these prognostic factors are surrogates for tumor biology; patients with more indolent tumors and oligometastatic burden have favorable prognosis.

Response to systemic therapy is an important consideration when selecting patients for metastasectomy. The ability to assess the patient's response to therapy and to make sure that no additional metastatic disease develops on treatment is the rationale for starting with systemic therapy rather than a surgery first approach, even with oligometastatic disease. He and colleagues[43] performed metastasectomy for isolated residual foci of metastatic disease, isolated progressive disease in the setting of stable disease elsewhere, or for symptomatic disease in patients who were treated with vemurafenib within 30 days of surgery. Patients who had a longer duration of treatment had improved survival compared with those who underwent surgery in a more urgent fashion (hazard ratio, 2.93). Faries and colleagues[44] recently showed improved overall survival among patients who had an objective response or stable disease on systemic therapy before hepatic metastasectomy. As a general principle, with effective immunotherapy and targeted agent utilization, surgical resection for metastatic disease can be considered for stable or responding oligometastatic lesions or isolated progressive lesions with stable disease elsewhere when curative resection is feasible.

- A long DFI, isolated sites of progressive disease, and objective response to modern therapy are important considerations for metastasectomy.

Metastasectomy by M1 Classification

The eighth edition of the American Joint Commission for Cancer guidelines contains 4 categories of M1 disease and is subclassified by serum lactate dehydrogenase levels[39](**Table 1**). M1a classification defines distant metastases to skin, soft tissue, or distant lymph nodes and represents 20% of all stage IV disease.[45] Data from the MSLT-1 showed that, among the 32 patients who underwent treatment of M1a metastases, patients with complete surgical resection had a median overall survival rate of 60 months compared with 12.4 months among those who underwent medical therapy alone.[11] Patients with nodal involvement, however, had worse outcomes compared with skin and soft tissue involvement.[5,46] Microscopically negative resection margins are acceptable for metastasectomy of M1a disease, as opposed to the gross 1- to

Table 1
Four categories of M1 disease and is subclassified by serum lactate dehydrogenase levels

Classification	Site	Lactate Dehydrogenase Value
M1a	Distant metastasis to skin, soft tissue	Not recorded or unspecified
M1a (0)	including muscle, and/or nonregional	Not elevated
M1a (1)	lymph node	Elevated
M1b	Distant metastasis to lung with or	Not recorded or unspecified
M1b (0)	without M1a sites of disease	Not elevated
M1b (1)		Elevated
M1c	Distant metastasis to noncentral nervous	Not recorded or unspecified
M1c (0)	system visceral sites with or without	Not elevated
M1c (1)	M1a or M1b sites of disease	Elevated
M1b	Distant metastasis to central nervous	Not recorded or unspecified
M1d (0)	system with or without M1a, M1b, or	Not elevated
M1d (1)	M1c sites of disease	Elevated

Data from Gershenwald JE, Scolyer RA, Hess KR, Sondak VK, Long GV, Ross MI, et al. Melanoma staging: Evidence-based changes in the American Joint Committee on Cancer eighth edition cancer staging manual. CA Cancer J Clin. 2017;67(6):472-92.

2-cm margins required for primary site wide local excision. Currently, FDA approval is granted for T-VEC oncolytic therapy for unresectable M1a disease. Neoadjuvant therapy trials using T-VEC are underway,[47] which may help to downstage tumor and improve resectability, ultimately improving surgical selection and outcomes for M1a disease. Neoadjuvant approaches using immune checkpoint inhibitors and BRAF/MEK inhibition are also being evaluated.[48,49]

Pulmonary metastasis (M1b) is the most common category of M1 disease, representing up to 42% of patients with stage IV melanoma, and has a better prognosis than visceral involvement.[40,45] When clinical factors reflective of tumor biology are considered and complete resection of pulmonary involvement is feasible, the median survival after pulmonary metastasectomy ranges from 11 months to 40 months, with up to a 31% overall survival rate at 5 years.[46,50] Patients who do not undergo resection have median survivals of 6 to 13 months and a 0% to 4% overall survival rate at 5 years.[9] Patient selection is critical, with particular consideration given for DFI, the number of pulmonary lesions, and presence of extrathoracic disease.[9] Fortunately, high-resolution imaging has allowed for improved surveillance and staging of the burden of disease, which has been associated with improved outcomes after metastasectomy.[51] Durable long-term survival is possible, but is predicated on complete resection of metastatic disease.[52]

Under the current American Joint Commission for Cancer guidelines, M1c disease includes distant metastases to non–central nervous system visceral sites with or without M1a or M1b sites of disease. Before immunotherapy, 5-year overall survival rates of 38% to 41% have been reported for M1c disease.[9,53] When appropriately selected, adrenal metastasectomy has shown improved median survival of 20 to 25 months.[54,55] Similar outcomes have been reported for hepatic metastasectomy.[44] Central nervous system involvement, or M1d disease, occurs in up to 50% of patients with stage IV disease and results in up to 54% of the deaths from melanoma.[56,57] Most commonly, these lesions are symptomatic,[57] and surgery is often combined with whole-brain radiation or stereotactic radiotherapy because it may improve neurologic symptoms and improve survival.[56,57] Patients who underwent surgery and radiation had a median overall survival of 8.9 months, whereas the median survival for supportive care alone was 2.1 months.[58]

Outcomes in the Modern Era

Although data regarding metastasectomy in the current immunotherapy era are sparse, a recent study from Memorial Sloan Kettering evaluated patient outcomes after metastasectomy after immune checkpoint therapy.[59] This valuable study included a cohort of 237 highly selected patients with advanced stage III and stage IV melanoma. For all patients, among whom 88% had stage IV disease, the estimated 5-year survival was 75%. Of those who had stable disease or disease responsive to immune checkpoint therapy (n = 12), survival approached 90%. Those with isolated sites of progression who underwent resection (n = 106) had a 60% 5-year overall survival rate. The median survival was not reached in either group. Those who had multifocal progression (n = 119) and underwent palliative resection did significantly worse, with a median overall survival of 7.8 months.[9] This study provides promising evidence for the role of metastasectomy with effective and durable systemic immunotherapy treatments.

- In the era of modern effective therapy, the 5-year overall survival has been estimated at 75% in a cohort study using immune checkpoint therapy and selective metastasectomy.

MESTASTASECTOMY AS AN ADJUNCT TO SYSTEMIC THERAPY: ADOPTIVE CELL THERAPY

Current systemic immunotherapies activate and enhance host immune responses. Adoptive cell therapy represents a new shift in highly personalized cancer therapy that directly delivers tumor-reactive lymphocytes into the host and can result in durable complete responses in melanoma.[60] Surgically resected melanoma tumor deposits are processed and cultured with high-dose IL-2 to expand tumor-infiltrating lymphocytes (TIL).[61] TIL with sufficient growth and anti-tumor reactivity are selectively expanded. This process may take 6 weeks, but will produce up to 10^{11} lymphocytes.[60] The patient is then lymphodepleted with aggressive chemotherapy and the expanded TIL are infused. TIL expansion is stimulated by high-dose IL-2.[61]

Unlike conventional forms of immunotherapy that rely on the host for production of sufficient immune cells, this therapy grows antitumor lymphocytes in vitro, selects cells with the highest avidity for tumor specific antigens, and can be activated in vitro so that these cells may overcome in vivo inhibition.[60] Until recently, this technique was not available outside of the National Cancer Institute, where objective response rates approached 55% with a 22% durable response.[60] The brain is not a sanctuary site with TIL therapy; therefore, patients with brain metastases are potentially eligible for this therapy and responses have been reported.[62]

The surgeon's role in an adoptive cell therapy program is to assist with resection of metastases for TIL harvest. The best TIL targets are those that can be safely resected with minimal risk of complications that allow the patient to undergo the aggressive immunoablative regimen necessary for TIL reinfusion and expansion. Superficial subcutaneous metastases or lymph node metastases in the cervical, axillary, or inguinal distribution are examples of good targets for TIL harvest. The operation should be as minimally invasive as possible. Brain metastases or hollow viscus metastases (ie, bowel metastases) are not ideal TIL harvest targets owing to issues related to recovery and contamination of the specimen.

- Surgery in metastatic patients can also be used to improve therapeutic options for systemic therapy.
- Obtaining tissue in a safe and reasonable manner allows patients to potentially undergo adoptive cell therapy.

PALLIATIVE SURGERY

The typical focus of surgical oncology is related to long-term survival. However, relief of patient suffering remains a critical role for the surgeon, particularly for patients with metastatic disease. Patients with unresectable disease or unfavorable tumor biology have worse overall survival, but surgery can provide excellent palliation when the expectations of surgical goals are understood and met. Ultimately, providing patients with maintenance of their quality of life is imperative and patients may benefit from surgical palliation. Symptoms from locally advanced metastatic tumors may prevent a patient from undergoing systemic therapy, and palliation in this regard may ultimately provide an opportunity to receive effective systemic therapy. Surgery should be accomplished with minimal morbidity and length of hospital stay. The focus should be to alleviate specific symptoms such as bleeding or intestinal obstruction.[63] With these goals in mind, surgical palliation may provide relief in 77% to 100% of patients.[64] Ollila and colleagues[53] showed that 97% of patients had relief after resections of gastrointestinal obstructions. With the intent of palliation of symptoms, surgery will remain an integral component of management of the patient with advanced melanoma.

- Surgical palliation will always play a critical role in the management of metastatic patients to relieve suffering for symptoms such as bleeding or intestinal obstruction.

SUMMARY

Before immune therapy and oncolytic therapy, only very modest survival gains were achieved with metastasectomy.[5] With more effective systemic therapies achieving durable responses approaching 40%,[24,25] surgery can be used in patients selected to have more favorable tumor biology. Indeed, in this setting, recent evidence has been very promising with 5-year overall survival of 75% in patients with advanced melanoma.[59] Optimal treatment sequencing remains to be defined and is a matter of current debate and investigation.[9,43,59] Surgery, however, will remain an essential component of the multidisciplinary management of metastatic melanoma.

DISCLOSURE

K.M. McMasters: Scientific Advisory Board, Elucida Oncology. The remaining authors have nothing to disclose.

REFERENCES

1. American Cancer Society. Cancer facts & figures 2019. Atlanta (GA): American Cancer Society; 2019.
2. Siegel RL, Miller KD, Jemal A. Cancer statistics, 2018. CA Cancer J Clin 2018; 68(1):7–30.
3. Morton DL, Thompson JF, Cochran AJ, et al. Final trial report of sentinel-node biopsy versus nodal observation in melanoma. N Engl J Med 2014;370(7):599–609.

4. Barth A, Wanek LA, Morton DL. Prognostic factors in 1,521 melanoma patients with distant metastases. J Am Coll Surg 1995;181(3):193–201.

5. Karakousis CP, Velez A, Driscoll DL, et al. Metastasectomy in malignant melanoma. Surgery 1994;115(3):295–302.

6. Ollila DW, Hsueh EC, Stern SL, et al. Metastasectomy for recurrent stage IV melanoma. J Surg Oncol 1999;71(4):209–13.

7. Sondak VK, Liu PY, Warneke J, et al. Surgical resection for stage IV melanoma: A Southwest Oncology Group trial (S9430). J Clin Oncol. 2006;24(18_suppl):8019.

8. Faries MB, Mozzillo N, Kashani-Sabet M, et al. Long-term survival after complete surgical resection and adjuvant immunotherapy for distant melanoma metastases. Ann Surg Oncol 2017;24(13):3991–4000.

9. Bello DM. Indications for the surgical resection of stage IV disease. J Surg Oncol 2019;119(2):249–61.

10. Agrawal S, Yao TJ, Coit DG. Surgery for melanoma metastatic to the gastrointestinal tract. Ann Surg Oncol 1999;6(4):336–44.

11. Howard JH, Thompson JF, Mozzillo N, et al. Metastasectomy for distant metastatic melanoma: analysis of data from the first Multicenter Selective Lymphadenectomy Trial (MSLT-I). Ann Surg Oncol 2012;19(8):2547–55.

12. Postow MA, Chesney J, Pavlick AC, et al. Nivolumab and ipilimumab versus ipilimumab in untreated melanoma. N Engl J Med 2015;372(21):2006–17.

13. Long GV, Hauschild A, Santinami M, et al. Adjuvant Dabrafenib plus Trametinib in Stage III BRAF-mutated melanoma. N Engl J Med 2017;377(19):1813–23.

14. Hodi FS, Chiarion-Sileni V, Gonzalez R, et al. Nivolumab plus ipilimumab or nivolumab alone versus ipilimumab alone in advanced melanoma (CheckMate 067): 4-year outcomes of a multicentre, randomised, phase 3 trial. Lancet Oncol 2018; 19(11):1480–92.

15. Serrone L, Zeuli M, Sega FM, et al. Dacarbazine-based chemotherapy for metastatic melanoma: thirty-year experience overview. J Exp Clin Cancer Res 2000; 19(1):21–34.

16. Hill GJ 2nd, Krementz ET, Hill HZ. Dimethyl triazeno imidazole carboxamide and combination therapy for melanoma. IV. Late results after complete response to chemotherapy (Central Oncology Group protocols 7130, 7131, and 7131A). Cancer 1984;53(6):1299–305.

17. Chapman PB, Einhorn LH, Meyers ML, et al. Phase III multicenter randomized trial of the Dartmouth regimen versus dacarbazine in patients with metastatic melanoma. J Clin Oncol 1999;17(9):2745–51.

18. Atkins MB, Lotze MT, Dutcher JP, et al. High-dose recombinant interleukin 2 therapy for patients with metastatic melanoma: analysis of 270 patients treated between 1985 and 1993. J Clin Oncol 1999;17(7):2105–16.

19. Atkins MB, Hsu J, Lee S, et al. Phase III trial comparing concurrent biochemotherapy with cisplatin, vinblastine, dacarbazine, interleukin-2, and interferon alfa-2b with cisplatin, vinblastine, and dacarbazine alone in patients with metastatic malignant melanoma (E3695): a trial coordinated by the Eastern Cooperative Oncology Group. J Clin Oncol 2008;26(35):5748–54.

20. Keilholz U, Punt CJ, Gore M, et al. Dacarbazine, cisplatin, and interferon-alfa-2b with or without interleukin-2 in metastatic melanoma: a randomized phase III trial (18951) of the European Organisation for Research and Treatment of Cancer Melanoma Group. J Clin Oncol 2005;23(27):6747–55.

21. Eton O, Legha SS, Bedikian AY, et al. Sequential biochemotherapy versus chemotherapy for metastatic melanoma: results from a phase III randomized trial. J Clin Oncol 2002;20(8):2045–52.

22. Ives NJ, Stowe RL, Lorigan P, et al. Chemotherapy compared with bio-chemotherapy for the treatment of metastatic melanoma: a meta-analysis of 18 trials involving 2,621 patients. J Clin Oncol 2007;25(34):5426–34.

23. Hodi FS, O'Day SJ, McDermott DF, et al. Improved survival with ipilimumab in patients with metastatic melanoma. N Engl J Med 2010;363(8):711–23.

24. Robert C, Schachter J, Long GV, et al. Pembrolizumab versus Ipilimumab in advanced melanoma. N Engl J Med 2015;372(26):2521–32.

25. Robert C, Long GV, Brady B, et al. Nivolumab in previously untreated melanoma without BRAF mutation. N Engl J Med 2015;372(4):320–30.

26. Weber J, Mandala M, Del Vecchio M, et al. Adjuvant Nivolumab versus Ipilimumab in resected Stage III or IV melanoma. N Engl J Med 2017;377(19):1824–35.

27. Chapman PB, Hauschild A, Robert C, et al. Improved survival with vemurafenib in melanoma with BRAF V600E mutation. N Engl J Med 2011;364(26):2507–16.

28. Robert C, Karaszewska B, Schachter J, et al. Improved overall survival in melanoma with combined dabrafenib and trametinib. N Engl J Med 2015;372(1):30–9.

29. Ribas A, Gonzalez R, Pavlick A, et al. Combination of vemurafenib and cobimetinib in patients with advanced BRAF(V600)-mutated melanoma: a phase 1b study. Lancet Oncol 2014;15(9):954–65.

30. Long GV, Menzies AM, Nagrial AM, et al. Prognostic and clinicopathologic associations of oncogenic BRAF in metastatic melanoma. J Clin Oncol 2011;29(10): 1239–46.

31. Hauschild A, Grob JJ, Demidov LV, et al. Dabrafenib in BRAF-mutated metastatic melanoma: a multicentre, open-label, phase 3 randomised controlled trial. Lancet 2012;380(9839):358–65.

32. Puzanov I, Milhem MM, Minor D, et al. Talimogene Laherparepvec in combination with ipilimumab in previously untreated, unresectable stage IIIB-IV melanoma. J Clin Oncol 2016;34(22):2619–26.

33. Kaufman HL, Ruby CE, Hughes T, et al. Current status of granulocyte-macrophage colony-stimulating factor in the immunotherapy of melanoma. J Immunother Cancer 2014;2:11.

34. Liu BL, Robinson M, Han ZQ, et al. ICP34.5 deleted herpes simplex virus with enhanced oncolytic, immune stimulating, and anti-tumour properties. Gene Ther 2003;10(4):292–303.

35. Goldsmith K, Chen W, Johnson DC, et al. Infected cell protein (ICP)47 enhances herpes simplex virus neurovirulence by blocking the CD8+ T cell response. J Exp Med 1998;187(3):341–8.

36. Andtbacka RH, Kaufman HL, Collichio F, et al. Talimogene Laherparepvec improves durable response rate in patients with advanced melanoma. J Clin Oncol 2015;33(25):2780–8.

37. Chesney J, Puzanov I, Collichio F, et al. Randomized, open-label phase II study evaluating the efficacy and safety of talimogene laherparepvec in combination with ipilimumab versus ipilimumab alone in patients with advanced, unresectable melanoma. J Clin Oncol 2018;36(17):1658–67.

38. Andtbacka RHI, Dummer R, Gyorki DE, et al. Interim analysis of a randomized, open-label phase 2 study of talimogene laherparepvec (T-VEC) neoadjuvant treatment (neotx) plus surgery (surgx) vs surgx for resectable stage IIIB-IVM1a melanoma (MEL). J Clin Oncol. 2018;36(15_suppl):9508.

39. Gershenwald JE, Scolyer RA, Hess KR, et al. Melanoma staging: evidence-based changes in the American Joint Committee on Cancer eighth edition cancer staging manual. CA Cancer J Clin 2017;67(6):472–92.

40. Essner R, Lee JH, Wanek LA, et al. Contemporary surgical treatment of advanced-stage melanoma. Arch Surg 2004;139(9):961–6 [discussion: 6–7].

41. Ollila DW, Stern SL, Morton DL. Tumor doubling time: a selection factor for pulmonary resection of metastatic melanoma. J Surg Oncol 1998;69(4):206–11.

42. Ollila DW. Complete metastasectomy in patients with stage IV metastatic melanoma. Lancet Oncol 2006;7(11):919–24.

43. He M, Lovell J, Ng BL, et al. Post-operative survival following metastasectomy for patients receiving BRAF inhibitor therapy is associated with duration of pre-operative treatment and elective indication. J Surg Oncol 2015;111(8):980–4.

44. Faries MB, Leung A, Morton DL, et al. A 20-year experience of hepatic resection for melanoma: is there an expanding role? J Am Coll Surg 2014;219(1):62–8.

45. Balch CM, Gershenwald JE, Soong SJ, et al. Final version of 2009 AJCC melanoma staging and classification. J Clin Oncol 2009;27(36):6199–206.

46. Ollila DW, Gleisner AL, Hsueh EC. Rationale for complete metastasectomy in patients with stage IV metastatic melanoma. J Surg Oncol 2011;104(4):420–4.

47. Andtbacka RHI, Chastain M, Li A, et al. Phase 2, multicenter, randomized, open label trial assessing efficacy and safety of talimogene laherparepvec (T-VEC) neoadjuvant treatment (tx) plus surgery vs surgery for resectable stage IIIB/C and IVM1a melanoma (MEL). J Clin Oncol. 2015;33(15_suppl). TPS9094-TPS.

48. Blankenstein SA, Rohaan MW, Klop WMC, et al. Neoadjuvant cytoreductive treatment with BRAF/MEK inhibition of prior unresectable regionally advanced melanoma to allow complete surgical resection: REDUCTOR trial. J Clin Oncol. 2019;37(15_suppl):9587.

49. Rozeman EA, Blank CU, Akkooi ACJV, et al. Neoadjuvant ipilimumab 1 nivolumab (IPI1NIVO) in palpable stage III melanoma: updated data from the OpACIN trial and first immunological analyses. J Clin Oncol. 2017;35(15_suppl):9586.

50. Leo F, Cagini L, Rocmans P, et al. Lung metastases from melanoma: when is surgical treatment warranted? Br J Cancer 2000;83(5):569–72.

51. Dalrymple-Hay MJ, Rome PD, Kennedy C, et al. Pulmonary metastatic melanoma – the survival benefit associated with positron emission tomography scanning. Eur J Cardiothorac Surg 2002;21(4):611–4 [discussion: 4–5].

52. Petersen RP, Hanish SI, Haney JC, et al. Improved survival with pulmonary metastasectomy: an analysis of 1720 patients with pulmonary metastatic melanoma. J Thorac Cardiovasc Surg 2007;133(1):104–10.

53. Ollila DW, Essner R, Wanek LA, et al. Surgical resection for melanoma metastatic to the gastrointestinal tract. Arch Surg 1996;131(9):975–9, 9-80.

54. Haigh PI, Essner R, Wardlaw JC, et al. Long-term survival after complete resection of melanoma metastatic to the adrenal gland. Ann Surg Oncol 1999;6(7):633–9.

55. Mittendorf EA, Lim SJ, Schacherer CW, et al. Melanoma adrenal metastasis: natural history and surgical management. Am J Surg 2008;195(3):363–8 [discussion: 8–9].

56. Sampson JH, Carter JH Jr, Friedman AH, et al. Demographics, prognosis, and therapy in 702 patients with brain metastases from malignant melanoma. J Neurosurg 1998;88(1):11–20.

57. Leung AM, Hari DM, Morton DL. Surgery for distant melanoma metastasis. Cancer J 2012;18(2):176–84.

58. Fife KM, Colman MH, Stevens GN, et al. Determinants of outcome in melanoma patients with cerebral metastases. J Clin Oncol 2004;22(7):1293–300.

59. Bello DM, Panageas KS, Hollmann TJ, et al. Outcomes of patients with metastatic melanoma selected for surgery after immunotherapy (Abstract 5). Society of Surgical Oncology Annual Cancer Symposium. 2018.
60. Rosenberg SA, Restifo NP. Adoptive cell transfer as personalized immunotherapy for human cancer. Science 2015;348(6230):62–8.
61. Klemen ND, Feingold PL, Goff SL, et al. Metastasectomy following immunotherapy with adoptive cell transfer for patients with advanced melanoma. Ann Surg Oncol 2017;24(1):135–41.
62. Hong JJ, Rosenberg SA, Dudley ME, et al. Successful treatment of melanoma brain metastases with adoptive cell therapy. Clin Cancer Res 2010;16(19): 4892–8.
63. Allen PJ, Coit DG. The surgical management of metastatic melanoma. Ann Surg Oncol 2002;9(8):762–70.
64. Wornom IL 3rd, Smith JW, Soong SJ, et al. Surgery as palliative treatment for distant metastases of melanoma. Ann Surg 1986;204(2):181–5.

Moving?

Make sure your subscription moves with you!

To notify us of your new address, find your **Clinics Account Number** (located on your mailing label above your name), and contact customer service at:

Email: journalscustomerservice-usa@elsevier.com

800-654-2452 (subscribers in the U.S. & Canada)
314-447-8871 (subscribers outside of the U.S. & Canada)

Fax number: 314-447-8029

Elsevier Health Sciences Division
Subscription Customer Service
3251 Riverport Lane
Maryland Heights, MO 63043

*To ensure uninterrupted delivery of your subscription, please notify us at least 4 weeks in advance of move.